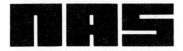

NURSES' AIDS SERIES

Paediatric Nursing

Sixth Edition

Barbara F. Weller
RSCN, SRN, RNT
Nursing Officer, Department of Health, Elephant & Castle, London

Sheila Barlow
RSCN, SRN, RNT
Director of Nurse Education, The Hospitals for Sick Children, Charles West School of Nursing, 24 Great Ormond Street, London

Baillière Tindall **London Philadelphia Toronto**

Baillière Tindall   1 St Anne's Road
W. B. Saunders   Eastbourne, East Sussex BN21 3UN, England

West Washington Square
Philadelphia, PA 19105, USA

1 Goldthorne Avenue
Toronto, Ontario M8Z 5T9, Canada

Apartado 26370—Cedro 512
Mexico 4, DF Mexico

Rua Evaristo da Veiga, 55, 20° andar
Rio de Janeiro — RJ, Brazil

ABP Australia Ltd, 44–50 Waterloo Road
North Ryde, NSW 2113, Australia

Ichibancho Central Building, 22–1 Ichibancho
Chiyoda-ku, Tokyo 102, Japan

10/fl, Inter-Continental Plaza, 94 Granville Road
Tsim Sha Tsui East, Kowloon, Hong Kong

First published 1961
Sixth edition 1983
   Reprinted 1985

Printed in Great Britain by
William Clowes Limited, Beccles and London

British Library Cataloguing in Publication Data
Weller, Barbara F.
   Paediatric Nursing.—6th ed.—(Nurses' aids series)
   1. Paediatric nursing
   I. Title   II. Barlow, Sheila   III. Series
   610.73'62   RJ 245
ISBN 0-7020-1013-8

Contents

Preface

A child cured of meningitis but who was left blind, deaf, spastic and apparently mindless was heard by the Ward Sister to say 'one–two–three–four' when playing with some toys which she had persisted in providing. He later went on to recovery and to be educated. The Ward Sister, Miss Duncombe, went on to achieve a high position in paediatric nursing and wrote the first editions of *Paediatric Nursing* in the Nurses' Aids Series; a book used and valued by thousands of nurses in many countries. The current authors have therefore inherited a proud tradition and a considerable challenge in the re-writing of this new edition which will be the first without Miss Duncombe's involvement, although she has provided much valued encouragement.

Miss Sheila Barlow, Director of Nurse Education, is welcomed to the author partnership. Miss Barlow brings considerable expertise and experience to this textbook which is based on the educational needs of many thousands of student nurses.

Paediatric nursing is a rapidly expanding speciality. Nurses must be able to meet the technological changes in intensive care areas and also be well informed of developments in the primary health care services in the community affecting the child and the family. The paediatric nurse also needs to be well read, and sensitive in matters pertaining to the emotional well being of the children and their families about whose care she is concerned.

The gathering together of all these aspects in *Paediatric*

Nursing will enable the student nurse reader to enhance the quality of care she is concerned with giving to the children with the help of qualified staff. The student nurse working in the children's ward for the first time is often perplexed and puzzled by what she finds—the organized chaos, the unusual routines, the noise and parental involvement in care. It is often difficult for her to relate this environment to the new paediatric nursing knowledge she is seeking to acquire.

The authors hope that this sixth edition of *Paediatric Nursing* will provide the reader with a basis or framework with which she can pursue her paediatric experience in a logical and meaningful manner. In keeping with the Nursing Process concept, a problem-solving approach has been used in many areas whilst retaining the essentially practical nature of the text.

Acknowledgements

We would like to thank friends and colleagues for their valuable suggestions and comments. Very special thanks are due to Miss Elaine Morgan, Clinical Nurse Teacher, The Hospitals for Sick Children, for her energy, enthusiasm and persistence in seeing to the organization of all the illustrations.

Several of the old and new illustrations are taken from the files of the Department of Medical Illustration, Institute of Child Health, The Hospitals for Sick Children, and we should like to thank Mr R. J. Lunnon, FIIP, FRCPS and Mr M. Johns for these and also for their kind assistance. We should also like to acknowledge the new illustrations (Figs 9, 26) provided by Vickers Medical Ltd, also Wyeth Ltd who provided illustration No. 7.

1983   Sheila Barlow
                                                  Barbara F. Weller

Part I
Basic principles of paediatric nursing

1 The healthy child

An understanding of the normal development of the child, together with her own observations will enable the nurse to provide care for sick children that recognizes and meets the child's individual needs. No two children are alike and the norms and milestones of average development must never be taken too literally. Each child is a unique individual.

Children do not exist in isolation but have parents (or parent substitutes) and are members of families with their own differing social and cultural influences. The nurse's assessment also needs to recognize that the environment, previous life experiences, family and home will all have important implications for the individual child's development and growth, both physical, mental and emotional.

The average standards are known as norms or milestones. They should be familiar to those who deal with children both in health and sickness, but it is important to realize that variations of up to 10 or 15% below or above any of these standards may still be considered within normal limits. For this reason, many paediatricians now refer to developmental progress as a percentile of the average, rather than using rigid figures.

ANTENATAL CARE

Good antenatal care is important to the future development of the child. Attendance by the mother at the maternity clinic at regular intervals during pregnancy will ensure that any problems which may influence fetal development are recognized promptly, as well as providing an opportunity for the mother (and father) to attend parentcraft sessions, e.g. in breast-feeding, in order to help the parents rear their baby happily and successfully.

FETAL DEVELOPMENT

Development of the fetus during pregnancy is a time of rapid growth. After fertilization, when the spermatozoon meets an ovum usually in the outer third of the Fallopian tube, the cells multiply rapidly into a morula which passes into the uterine cavity and embeds in the endometrium.

After 4 weeks the fetal shape resembles a mammal and is about 1 cm long. By about 8 weeks limbs have developed. At 12 weeks the fetus is obviously human and the external genitalia will reveal the sex. The length is now about 9 cm. All essential organs have formed before the twelfth week. After this the fetus continues to grow and at about the 27/28th week the fetus is said to be viable. i.e. if born the fetus attempts to breathe. After 28 weeks the fetal muscles develop and fat is laid down. The fetus is coated with a greasy substance known as vernix. The fetus is now able to move quite freely within the amniotic cavity.

THE CHILD AT BIRTH

The average newborn infant may be expected to weigh approximately 3.5 kg (7½ lb) and to be about 50 cm (20 in.) long. The head circumference is approximately 33 cm (13 in.) with a cranium which is disproportionately large compared with the face.

Anterior and posterior fontanelles are open, moulding may be present and the sutures can be felt. The limbs seem short in comparison with the body, and the head and abdomen large in comparison with the thorax. Subcutaneous fat is sparse, the skin looks red and elastic and the hair is, as a rule, merely a fine down-like growth. The nails are soft and are inclined to peel off. The eyes lack pigment and usually appear blue. Reaction to light is merely reflex. Hearing is present. The infant is sensitive to hot and cold and responds to pain and hunger. Movements are mostly reflex. The respiratory rate is rapid at 40 breaths/min and is frequently irregular in rhythm. The heat regulating centre is immature and variations in the body temperature may be sudden and considerable.

At birth, the newborn infant is utterly dependent on the adults around him. He is aware of changes in temperature, of being touched and of being handled, of sounds and of bright lights. He sleeps for long periods, crys, sucks and can make discriminating sounds.

Various reflexes are present. The main ones are:

1. Pupil reflexes—the newborn infant will turn his head towards the source of light providing it is not too bright. In pre-term babies the light may need to be shone for a longer period before this reflex is obtained.

2. Moro reflex—response to sudden sound causing the infant's body to stiffen, the arms to go up and out, then forward and towards each other. This reflex usually disappears at about the age of 3–4 months and may be difficult to elicit in the pre-term infant.

3. The grasp reflex—this may be obtained in the hand or foot by either introducing a finger into the palm of the hand which the infant grasps quite strongly or by gently stroking the sole of the foot behind the toes.

4. Placing and walking reflexes—obtained by holding the infant upright over the edge of a table, so that the sole of the foot presses against the edge. The infant will bend his hips and knees, putting the foot on the table. The opposite foot 'steps' forward.

5. Withdrawal reflex—pricking the sole of the foot will result in the infant's leg being flexed at the hip, knee and ankle.

6. Babinski's sign—stroking the sole of the foot causes the great toe to flex and the toes to fan out.

7. Rooting reflex—when the corner of the mouth is touched with a finger which moves towards the cheek, the infant will turn his head towards the object and open his mouth.

8. Asymmetrical tonic neck reflex—when the infant is lying quietly supine, the head may be turned to one side with the arm extended on the same side. The opposite knee is often flexed. This reflex usually disappears at about 2–3 months of age, but may persist longer and be more marked in spastic babies.

Developmental considerations for nursing care and play activities

Mothers and fathers should be encouraged to spend as much time as possible with their newborn infants, particularly during the first few hours after delivery. Research has shown this to be the optimal period for 'bonding' or parent/child attachment. Bonding enhances the behavioural development of the child whilst helping to ensure that the parents are able to provide the care necessary for the infant's future. Facilities should always be available for the mother/father to be resident with their newborn infant.

Parents not able to have extensive close contact with their newborn infant in these early days should be encouraged to visit, handle, fondle and care for their infants as soon as they are able to do so. In the Intensive Care situation it would be necessary to support and guide the parents in doing this. By acting as the 'role model' the nurse will be able to show the parents how to make physical contact with their baby, e.g. by placing their hands through the incubator portholes. This increases the parents' self-confidence and skill at care-giving before the infant is discharged from hospital.

Always ensure that, providing the infant's condition allows it, the baby is held during feeding so that he can watch his mother's (or nurse's) face. Talk, rock, touch, kiss, sing and call him by name during his waking hours in the 'en face' position (when the eyes of the infant and of the care-giver are on the same visual plane). Place a bright, attractive but simple mobile within 12–18 in. (255–450 cm) of the line of vision.

As the newborn infant's temperature regulating system is not yet fully efficient, care should be taken to ensure that the environmental temperature is kept reasonably consistent at 21–24°C (70–75°F). Clothing should be light but adequate.

AT 3 MONTHS

Weight 5 kg (11¼ lb). Head now normal shape and growing rapidly in circumference. Posteria fontanelle closed. Begins to balance head when held in the sitting position. Limbs now well covered, the face round and the skin elastic. Second growth of hair replaces the initial down. The eyes have their permanent colour. Has achieved some coordination of eye movements and fixes on objects and may notice new surroundings.

Recognizes his mother, responds to her smile and smiles with pleasure. Plays with own hands and feet. Attempts to grasp rattles and soft toys. Sleeps 18–20 h/24 h. Babbles in a socially responsive manner. Enjoys sucking for its own pleasure and will purposely place hand in mouth to suck.

Developmental considerations for nursing care and play activities

Opportunities for the infant to experience new sensations and textures should be provided by changing the position of

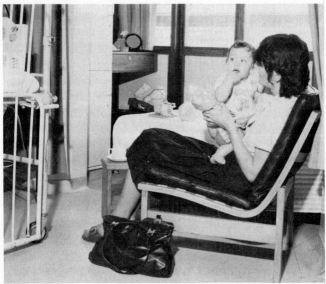

Fig. 1. Resident mother nursing sick infant.

the cot or moving the infant from a 'baby chair' to a mat on
the floor to allow full freedom of limb movements. Bathing
time can provide immense pleasure for the infant to enjoy
floating and splashing in the warm water.

Dangly toys should be suspended from the cot or pram,
within easy reach of the child's grasp. They should be
bright, of differing shades and textures, safely 'suckable'
and of a good hand size, yet, easy to clean and sterilize as
necessary. They should also be changed frequently to give
variety. Provide the infant with a rattle or other suitable
toys to hold in the hand, which are strong enough to sustain
dropping over the side of the cot.

The importance of the mother's presence to the infant
should be recognized and facilities provided for her (or for
a mother substitute) to be resident in hospital with her
child.

AT 6 MONTHS

Weight 7.5 kg (16½ lb). Eyes can follow people round; turns head to increase visual field. Can determine direction of sound. Enjoys new tastes and takes solid food. Begins to masticate and drink from a cup.

First teeth erupt (usually lower central incisors); carries everything to the mouth. Can hold objects in both hands. Grasps things deliberately. Sits up, if supported. Has pleasure in rocking his body. Spine is now very straight. Will smile at familiar faces and is capable of real laughter. Makes sounds involving the use of lips and tongue. Prepares for speech.

Becomes fretful if his mother disappears and may show fear and apprehension if strangers approach him.

Developmental considerations for nursing care and play activities

Involve mother/father actively in all care of the child. Always provide facilities for them to live in if they are able to do so. In the parents' absence, care should be provided by one or two nurses on an assignment basis. Consideration may be needed to adapt duty rosters to meet developmental needs.

Opportunities for outings in pram and for change of position from cot to high chair should be provided. Let the child participate in self-feeding at mealtimes with an extra spoon, finger held foods, etc.

The child enjoys repetitive games, e.g. 'Hide and Seek'. He enjoys, too, opportunities to bang and rattle objects which he is now able to transfer from one hand to the other, and will look for dropped toys if they fall over the side of the cot or pram. Nesting toys, cubes and squeezy toys are all suitable at this age. As everything still goes directly to the mouth, all toys should be small and easy to grasp, but not small enough to swallow.

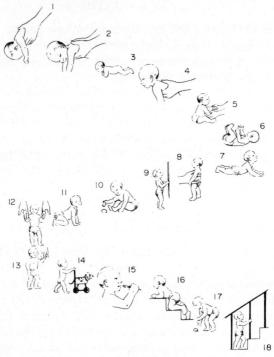

Fig. 2. Growth and motor development in the average child during the first 18 months. The figures indicate age in months.

AT THE END OF THE 1st YEAR

By this time the weight will be about 10.5 kg (23 lb), the length 73 cm (29 in.) and the head circumference 46 cm (18 in.). The face and the limbs are well covered with subcutaneous fat and there are dimples over the knuckles, elbows and knees. The skin is firm and elastic and no longer hangs in loose folds as in the newly born.

The toddler looks around freely. Lachrymation is now fully established and crying is accompanied by tears. The toddler is now able to eat most foods with the family, masticates well and is beginning to feed himself. He has between 10 and 12 teeth (central incisors, 4; lateral incisors, 4; premolars, 2–4). The hair may need its first cut and the nails are now strong and hard.

He sits up on his own, can move from one place to another and becomes expert in rolling from back to front and creeping, rolling and pushing himself along on his feet. He can pull himself up with the help of the bars of the cot or of a chair and makes ready for the first steps which he is likely to achieve some time between the age of 10–16 months.

During the latter part of the first year, the child enjoys movement skills of many kinds by constant experimenting. He can bring thumb and forefinger together and can pick up tiny objects. He loves tearing up paper. Most children can say several monosyllabic words, two or three proper words and may imitate a variety of sounds.

The toddler goes through a negative stage and may be quite difficult with diet for a time. When awake, the one-year-old is incredibly active but still needs 12–16 h of sleep every day. He is filled with curiosity and anxious to make contacts with others, provided strangers allow him to make their acquaintance slowly and approach him quietly. He still needs cuddling and close physical contact with his mother or other familiar person. The majority of children at this age have a precious 'cuddly', a teddy-bear or a soft doll.

Developmental considerations for nursing care and play activities

The toddler is still very reliant upon his mother (or mother substitute) and actively seeks her cooperation in play and other social activities. Enjoys pull-along and push toys as well as post-boxes and building bricks. Play is essentially self-directed, and attention span remains limited.

Allow every opportunity for movement but take care to provide a safe environment for the active inquisitive toddler in order to avoid accident.

He will enjoy being with other children, e.g. at mealtimes. Diet can now be more varied and he should be offered drinks from a cup. He may continue to suck from a bottle, especially on going to sleep or at times of stress.

AT 2 YEARS

Weight 11–12 kg. Height approximately half the anticipated adult height. First set of teeth is almost complete, 20 in all (central incisors, 4; lateral incisors, 4; premolars, 4, canines, 4; second molars, 4).

He has developed bladder control during the day and is beginning to for the night. Beginning to show signs of independence and emancipation. He is no longer wholly dependent on his mother and at this stage develops and exhibits a will of his own. Temper tantrums in response to frustration are common and, unless the child is wisely handled, this can prove a trying period for the family. The 2-year-old can usually say phrases of 3–4 words and has a vocabulary of approximately 900 words. He lives entirely in the present and mothering and affection are still very important. Family rituals are very important to him for his security, e.g. on going to bed at night or for his bathtime. The use of certain words, e.g. 'wee-wee' for micturition are also important to him. He continues to resent separation from his parents but is also showing an ability to handle separation for short periods at a time.

Developmental considerations for nursing care and play activities

Recognize that the child is still very dependent on his mother for security, but allow him opportunities to express his independence if able to do so. Encourage and support his parents to participate in nursing care and treatment.

All toys should be strong and suitable for the child's age. Such toys should include ordinary boxes, building-bricks, strong wooden engines and trucks, soft animals and glove-puppets. Sand, water and equipment which allows the child to imitate adult activities such as 'cooking', washing up, playing at 'doctors and nurses' and dressing up are all particularly popular. If any of the toys used can be taken apart, no part should be small enough for the child to swallow, inhale or to push into the nostrils or ears. He is now beginning to play simple games with other children and will enjoy the opportunity of being able to ride bicycles, trucks etc., if able to do so. He will also enjoy quiet moments when he can have simple story-books read to him.

AT 3 YEARS

Not growing at the same rapid rate. Physical shape changing from 'toddler chubbiness to school-age slenderness'. Incredibly active, he can jump off bottom steps and hop on one foot. Able to dress and undress himself if helped with buttons. Can brush his own teeth and wash face and hands if given some assistance. Able to build a tower of bricks.

Constantly asking questions and has a large vocabulary of approximately 1500 words. During this time, particularly if an only child, he may develop an imaginary companion or friend and tell 'tall stories' about their activities together.

Developmental considerations for nursing care and play activities

Recognize the child's abilities and provide opportunities for these skills to continue and develop, e.g. allow him to wash himself with some 'sideline' supervision. The presence of mother is still important to him but he is now able to accept separation for short periods. Facilities for parents to be resident are still required. Place in peer group in the ward. The child's 'imaginary friend' is part of normal development, and should be accepted without entering into the detail of the fantasy. Developing a keen sense of dramatic play, enjoys dressing up and acting out stories. Enjoys group activities and creative projects, e.g. making a collage mural for the ward noticeboard. Still likes a story-time, especially on going to bed.

AT 5–7 YEARS

Starting school. Growth is slower and steadier, with considerable variation between one child and another. The first teeth begin to disappear; permanent set commence erupting usually in the seventh year and proceed erupting at a rate of '4' a year until about the age of 14 years.

Very active, developing considerable coordination of fine muscle movements both in sports and manual dexterity.

Elementary reading/writing skills achieved at about the age of 6 years. Has a well-developed sense of time and of personal responsibility.

The family unit continues to be his main security, providing support and acceptance as he learns to cope with new major experiences. Many children experience 'negative phases', e.g. nail-biting, quarrelling, peevishness etc.; these episodes are, however, usually short-lived.

Developmental considerations for nursing care and play activities

Recognize that the child's apparent 'maturity' may break down during hospitalization. Reassure the child that he is not being babyish if he cries. Reassure the parents, too, that regression during times of sickness is normal. Encourage them to participate in care yet to recognize the child's growing need for independence.

Play activities should include group games as well as individual play. It may be necessary, sometimes, to gather the more mobile children around the bedside of a child confined to bed for activities such as 'story-time' or a game of 'pass the parcel'. Both boys and girls enjoy home-like activities: cooking, washing dolls' clothes, woodwork etc.

AT 8–11 YEARS

The slowed but gradual rate of growth is maintained during this period with progress towards future adult body shape. With the eruption of the permanent set of teeth, prophylactic dental care continues to be of importance.

A time of great energy in which the child pursues many physical activities and hobbies. Also a period of social-emotional growth which takes the child's experiences beyond that of his family. It is a time when the peer group which has its own norms (rules) outside the family is all important.

Developmental considerations for nursing care and play activities

Whenever possible see that the child is grouped with children of his own age and interests. Encourage his participation in treatment but recognize that there may be times/situations when the child needs to regress or 'divest' his apparent maturity. Always ensure that the parents are kept well-informed about treatment and progress. All the child's questions should be answered honestly and at a level which is appropriate to his understanding and language.

Group activities gain importance in play and the child should be given opportunities for organizing these. Acting out activities are less important whilst model building and group games such as 'ludo' are much more popular.

Television viewing is especially popular to this age group and will need some monitoring and supervision.

EARLY ADOLESCENCE

A period of transition leading up to puberty. Females attain puberty (menarche or the first period) about 1–2 years before the male. Both sexes are undergoing physical and emotional changes. The rate of growth shows considerable increase and it has been established that the timing of this growth spurt is related to the onset of puberty. Bodily changes and the appearance of secondary sex characteristics stimulate self-consciousness. Any deviations from members of the peer group will create anxiety and embarrassment to the individual child.

The pre-adolescent has enormous physical energy and a correpondingly healthy appetite with a consequent need for increased kilojoule (Calorie) intake.

ADOLESCENCE

The rapid growth in height and weight commences in early adolescence and continues until the adult body size is reached. Bone growth is completed in the female at about 18 years and in the male at about 20 years, marking the end of adolescence when biologically the body has reached maturity.

Of utmost importance to the adolescents are peer friendships which provide emotional support as well as assistance in the adolescent's search for personal identity. Family relationships may be strained at this time when parents often feel overwhelmed by their loss of authority and control of their child. The adolescent in turn may see his parents as being 'conservative or reactionary' representing the so-called 'generation gap'.

Developmental considerations for nursing care and play activities

The adolescent should be nursed in a separate ward for adolescents, or failing this in a cubicle or side room where the privacy is respected as far as is practical by the ward staff. Unless specifically requested it should always be out of bounds to the younger children in the ward.

Care should be taken to involve the adolescent in all discussions concerning his treatment and care. His opinions should be listened to and considered, and questions should be answered honestly and factually.

Friends from school/club/college should be encouraged to visit and join in any social activities. A record/cassette player should be provided (headphones may be necessary in view of the 'noise' of some modern 'pop' music). Whenever possible, snacks and drinks should be provided as a social activity for the adolescent and his friends, particularly if the adolescent is in hospital for some time. Opportunities, too, for hobbies to be pursued should be considered.

Some scheduling of visiting may be needed in order to avoid conflict of the young person's interests and of situations which may create stress and unnecessary anxiety, e.g. too many visitors at the same time. Care should be taken to keep parents informed about their child's treatment and progress.

Acceptance by the nursing staff of the young person's interests/clothes/appearance is important, although overt approval need not be given. Cigarette smoking may cause some conflict for the nursing staff in view of its health hazard. However, particularly if the young person has been smoking for some time, hospital is not the best place to forbid it. It would be better to provide set smoking times in private, and when the opportunities arise set a good example by refusing to smoke and also discussing with the adolescent the problems associated with smoking as a matter of health education.

EDUCATION

An important element of continuity in the life of all children is that of 'going to school' and thus becoming a member of the community outside his home and family. In the United Kingdom there is a statutory obligation for all children to be educated according to 'age, ability and aptitude'; local education authorities also have the power to provide facilities for home tuition and schooling in hospital.

Education in hospital

According to his condition, age and abilities, education should be continued for the sick child in hospital wherever possible. The schoolteacher provides a bridge between the normal school life at home and the hospital ward environment which is welcomed both by the parents and the children.

How this service is provided varies with each education authority. Some local education authorities provide education for children from the age of 2 years onwards and others may only appoint teachers on a part-time basis, whilst in hospitals where there is a large child population, a hospital school employing several teachers with its own head teacher may have been established.

In order to provide appropriately for the individual child, the schoolteacher should receive regular reports on the child's condition and have access to the nursing care plans.

The provision of nursing care will need to take into account the school programme, to avoid interruption as far as possible. The child's own school will usually cooperate to provide appropriate books, work and projects. Parents will often provide a willing 'ferrying service' between the child's own school and the hospital schoolteacher. This is particularly important for the older child worried about forthcoming examinations.

IMMUNIZATION AND VACCINATION

In the United Kingdom all immunization is voluntary and the Government relies on health education and personal contacts with family doctors and health visitors for the uptake of this service. Good knowledge of the advantages and possible dangers of immunization and vaccination, with a good personal approach, will set the minds of most mothers at rest and convince them of the value of these protective measures to the health of their children. It is possible to offer children substantive measures of protection against measles, diphtheria, whooping cough, tetanus and poliomyelitis. Also to protect young adolescent girls against the possibility of rubella in future pregnancies. The necessary injections can be given in the local Child Health Clinic, general practitioner's surgery and occasionally in the home by the family doctor or health visitor. It is usual to give three injections, at the ages of approximately 3, 5 and 9 months, respectively, to protect against diphtheria, tetanus and whooping cough. The poliomyelitis vaccine is given orally. Enforcement doses of polio, diphtheria and tetanus vaccines are recommended when the child starts school. It is useful to issue to every child a card which can be easily produced in case of accident, showing an up-to-date record of tetanus immunization and reinforcing injections.

Vaccination against measles is usually carried out during the 2nd year of life (measles is uncommon before the age of 12 months). One injection is sufficient and by that time immunization for diphtheria, tetanus and whooping cough will have been completed.

Diphtheria is now so little known in the United Kingdom that mothers who are ignorant of this disease frequently need some persuasion before they consent to immunization.

Rubella vaccine is now offered in one injection to young girls usually between the ages of 11 and 14 (about the time of the menarche). The dangers to the fetus, should a woman contract rubella during the first 3 months of pregnancy, are well known.

BCG vaccination against tuberculosis is not a routine procedure in the United Kingdom, but BCG (Bacillus Calmette-Guérin) is available to infants exposed to tuberculosis and to children who remain negative to tuberculosis testing at the age of 12–13 years. They can be given protection for several years by a BCG vaccine.

Further reading

ELKIND, D. & WEINER, I. B. (1978) *Development of the Child*. New York: Wiley.

General Nursing Council (1982) *Aspects of Sick Children's Nursing*, Section 1.

HOLT, K. S. (1977) *Developmental Paediatrics*. London: Butterworth.

ILLINGWORTH, R. S. (1980) *The Development of the Infant and Young Child*, 7th edn. London: Churchill Livingstone.

JENKINS, G. C. (1981) *The First Year of Life*. London: Churchill Livingstone.

Open University (1979) *The First Years of Life*. London: Ward Lock.

2 The newborn

This chapter is concerned with the first year of life, a period of rapid growth physically, mentally and socially that will never again be equalled. The infant is completely dependent on his parents or substitutes for survival.

Nursing care of an infant needs to be planned in relation to his clinical needs, his development and also his family situation. Shared care with parents enables the nurse to recognize the infant/parent special relationship and gives her an opportunity to provide the parental health education vital to the promotion of good health for the child's future.

Nursing newborn infants is a great responsibility at all times but even more so when they are pre-term, weak or sick. Changes in the infant's condition may be extremely sudden and of urgent importance, and the nurse must be observant and capable of fine judgement and swift action when caring for these babies.

General points

For the nursing of sick babies, the cot should be large enough to allow for all procedures to be carried out with ease and for adequate observation of the infant.

The majority of babies are best nursed lying flat. At the head end, the bottom sheet can be protected by a piece of plastic sheeting covered by a small pillow-case. This allows for easy and frequent change of linen if it becomes soiled by mucous secretions or vomit.

No baby under the age of one year should be given

ordinary pillows because of the possible danger of suffocation. In babies with dyspnoea or orthopnoea, or when it is
necessary to nurse the baby in a recumbent position, small
firm pillows may be built up in an armchair position or the
head of the mattress can be raised by placing a pillow
underneath it. Alternatively a baby 'Sitta' may be used to
nurse the baby comfortably and conveniently in the sitting
position. Babies who have to be nursed sitting upright, can
be held in position if a rolled up napkin is placed underneath
their thighs, under the draw sheet. It should always be
remembered that young babies should be allowed as much
freedom to move around and kick as is compatible with
their condition. They also like the stimulation of a change
in position whenever this is possible, e.g. if the infant is
nursed in the centre of a cubicle it may be a good idea to
move the cot adjacent to the window from time to time. The
opportunity to lie on a mat or rug on the floor to kick and
exercise will often be enjoyed.

Temperature recording

The safest and most accurate method for measuring an
infant's temperature is one that is taken rectally. Each
infant should have his own rectal thermometer which has a
short rounded bob usually coloured blue. Alternatively, an
electronic temperature probe or thermistor can be used,
which may be inserted into the rectum or oesophagus.
Low-reading thermometers should be used for all newborn,
pre-term, low birthweight and sick infants in order to
ensure the early recognition of hypothermia. A rectal
temperature is usually taken in all children up to the age of
one year unless otherwise indicated.

Method

When taking a rectal temperature the anal region is
cleansed and dried then the bulb of the thermometer is
inspected to ensure that it is intact and lubricated lightly

before being inserted approximately 2.5 cm (1 in.) into the rectum. The baby should be lying in his cot or on his mother's or the nurse's knee, his legs raised and the thermometer inserted and the buttocks held together with a thumb and finger each side whilst the thermometer is in place. Alternatively, the child may be placed in the left lateral position. The thermometer should be held in place for 1 min, then withdrawn, wiped on the corner of the baby's napkin and read. Rinse thermometer under a cold tap, shake down, dry and place in the thermometer container.

Taking the pulse and respirations

Both pulse and respirations are taken while the infant is asleep or resting and before he is disturbed or the cot-side lowered. In small infants it is often difficult to feel the radial pulse. Alternative methods are: feeling the pulse over the temporal artery immediately in front of the ear or over the external iliac or the femoral artery in the groin; or to count the pulsating movments of the fontanelle.

Record all temperature, pulse and respiration readings immediately onto the child's chart. Any sudden change, and all low/high temperatures should be reported to the nurse-in-charge.

Bathing a sick baby

In the United Kingdom most babies are bathed on the mother's or nurse's lap. Everything should be prepared and conveniently arranged before the baby is disturbed. The cubicle should be warm (21°C) and the windows closed. The nurse should wash her hands and observe the unit's protective technique. The temperature of the bathwater should be checked to feel comfortable to the nurse's elbow.

After taking the pulse and respirations the baby is lifted from his cot, his clothes taken off (but leaving his nappy on) and a bath towel securely wrapped around him. The nurse swabs his eyes with sterile cotton cool and water from within outwards, using each swab once only, dipped in a gallipot of tapwater. The nostrils and ears are cleaned and the face washed and dried. The temperature of the bath-water is rechecked. Holding the baby in the crook of the arm and supporting his head, the hair is washed and then dried. The nappy is removed and the buttocks cleaned—using wool swabs if necessary. If required, the temperature is taken. With a well-soaped hand, a lather is applied to the trunk and limbs. The baby is turned towards the nurse to lather the back. The baby is held securely and the head supported with the nurse's arm, then he is placed in the bath whilst retaining support. On lifting the baby out of the bath he is thoroughly dried, weighed if necessary and dressed. The cot is re-made, toys replaced and the cubicle tidied. The windows are opened if necessary, the curtains drawn back and the lid replaced on bin. Hands are washed and gown removed.

Requirements

Baby bath or suitable basin.

Face flannel.

Bath towels.

Nappies.

Clothes as required.

Toilet tray from locker.

Baby hair brush and nail scissors.

Bag of sterile wool swabs and gallipot.

Canvas cot.

Bins for soiled nappies and linen.

N.B. Clinical thermometer and lubricant and baby scales as required.

When discharging a baby home, the mother can be told that a daily bath is desirable but not essential and that it might well be omitted at her discretion should the only room available not be well heated at times.

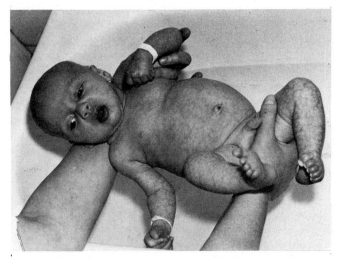

Fig. 3. A good way of holding a baby while lowering him into his bath.

Care of the umbilical cord

Following delivery, the cord is ligated to prevent haemor-rhage. The cord and ligature should be observed frequently for bleeding, stickiness, oozing or foul smell, all of which indicate infection and should be reported. Normally the cord becomes dry and necrosed within 5–10 days and falls off. The cord should be kept dry at all times. Occasionally triple dye or alcohol may be applied to promote drying.

Application of napkins

Increasingly, disposable napkins are being used; with some types special pants are worn. Whatever the type or method of putting the napkin on, in all cases the safety pin should lie horizontally in order to minimize any risk of injury should it accidentally become undone (Fig. 4).

Sore buttocks in the newborn may originate from a variety of causes, the most common of which are frequent loose

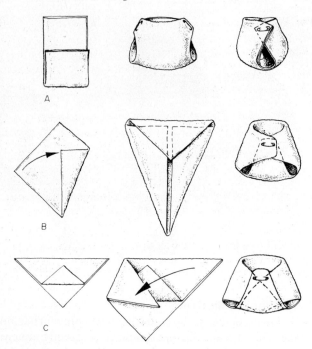

A

B

C

Fig. 4. Various ways of folding napkins.

stools, 'strong' ammoniacal urine, excessive fat in the feeds, careless or infrequent toilet and changes of napkins, inadequate rinsing of napkins after washing them in detergent, and unduly sensitive skin. Frequently the distribution of the rash gives a clue to the cause. A urine-soaked napkin will cause a widely distributed rash not only over the genitalia but spreading up to the abdomen and the sacrum and down to the thighs, while the skin folds and the natal cleft may be left unaffected. On the other hand, loose or fermented stools cause soreness of the perineum, around the anus and the back of the scrotum.

Intertrigo is a variant of napkin rash, which causes much soreness particularly in the groins and flexures. Intertrigo may also appear in the folds of the neck and is as a rule seen in fat and ill-kept babies. The soreness is caused by contact of two moist skin surfaces which are cut off from the air and gradually infected.

The *treatment of sore buttocks* varies according to the preference of those in charge and to the cause of the soreness. Dietary errors should be investigated and corrected. Ammonia dermatitis may be due either to a low fluid intake which is readily put right, or to decomposition of urine when in contact with stools and intestinal bacteria. Frequent changing and careful toilet is the best remedy.

In many cases it is a good idea to expose the infant's buttocks to the air, or wherever possible to the healing properties of sunlight. If this is done, the infant should wear bootees, and the feet may need light restraint using ankle restrainers.

The stools of the infant

The stools of the newborn infant are at first dark green to black in colour with a shiny appearance and viscid consistency, and are known as meconium. After 1–2 days they gradually change to lighter ones and are then called 'changing stools'. The stools of breast-fed babies are a golden mustard colour and of soft consistency. They have a characteristic, slightly sour smell. From one to six stools are passed each day.

The stools of infants fed on any type of infant formulae tend to be pale yellow, larger in bulk and more formed than those of breast-fed babies. From one to three stools are passed daily. The stools of infants should always be carefully observed, for much can be learned from their colour, odour, frequency and consistency. Changes occur readily and may be caused by slight deviation from health, change of the usual feed or amount of fluid intake, or by medicines.

It sometimes happens that a newborn baby fails to pass meconium in the first 24–36 hours. This is an important abnormality and must be reported at once as it may be due to a variety of serious causes such as imperforate anus, meconium ileus and atresia of the bowel.

PREVENTION OF INFECTION

Nursing procedures to prevent cross infection vary from unit to unit but the following principles will apply wherever infants are nursed.

1. Careful hand washing techniques by all members of the staff before touching an infant. This has been shown to be the single most important factor in reducing the spread of infection. Parents will need instruction in the techniques to be followed.

2. The correct technique in the use of gowns when used for infant care.

3. All staff should be free of respiratory, gastrointestinal or skin infections. If parents have an active infection they may need to be advised not to visit for a day or so. It might be suggested that a grandparent or aunt comes in their place whilst they are ill to avoid the risk of cross infection.

4. Each baby should have his own individual equipment including baby bath/basin.

5. All linen bins should have well-fitting seals/lids and be emptied at frequent and regular intervals.

6. All potential sources of infection, e.g. suction bottles, vaporizers etc., should be disinfected and changed regularly.

7. Liaison with the Infection Control Nurse and regular surveillance to monitor any reported infection.

8. Isolation procedures should be instigated imme-

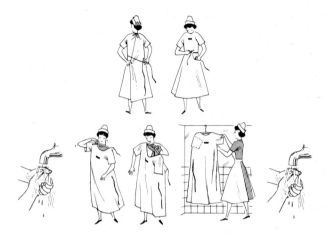

Fig. 5. Correct technique with barrier gowns.

diately with any sign or suspicion of infection. Preferably, the nurse caring for these infants would not be involved in the care of others. Parents will need support and guidance in the protocols to be followed in the isolation of their infants.

INFANT FEEDING

The normal infant approximately doubles his weight in the first 5 months of life and trebles his weight in the first year. In order to meet the demand for this rapid growth rate, the nutritional requirements of protein, carbohydrate, fats, vitamins, minerals and fluids must be met either by breast-feeding or by artificial feeding.

Breast-feeding

The best food for babies is undoubtedly human milk. All mothers should be encouraged to breast-feed their babies for a minimum of 2 weeks and preferably for the first 4–6 months.

Good reasons for breast-feeding

1. Protection against infection and allergies. Colostrum secreted in the first few days after birth is a rich source of antibodies. Breast-fed babies are less liable to gastrointestinal infections.

2. Human milk is rich in polyunsaturated fatty acids which are better absorbed by the infant than the fats in cows' milk.

3. There is no risk of giving an overconcentrated feed to the infant.

4. If sufficient breast milk is given the infant will not develop protein malnutrition. In developing countries, breast-feeding offers the only chance of survival for many infants.

In order for breast-feeding to be a success it is important that the details of breast-feeding are discussed with the parents antenatally. Good teaching and patience on the part of midwives and health visitors will also be required during pregnancy and postnatally for breast-feeding to become well-established. This may take as long as 14 days, during which time the mother may become anxious and so worried as to give up the attempt.

Undue stress on the importance of breast-feeding may, however, cause feelings of guilt if the mother is unable to manage this for any reason. The nurse, midwife or health visitor advising the mother should know the family circumstances and whatever the mother's choice for feeding she should be well-supported with advice and guidance.

Management of breast-feeding

Immediately after birth, the mother should cuddle her newborn infant to her breasts for about 15 min and allow the baby to suckle for 1 or 2 min at each breast if she intends to breast-feed. Suckling and cuddling the baby at this early stage is valuable psychologically, allowing mother and

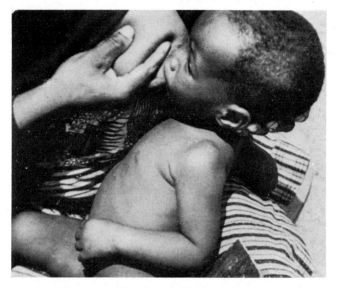

Fig. 6. Feeding position. The baby is held snugly against his mother with his head supported and his hands free. The nipple is guided by the fore and middle fingers (thumb and forefinger are also suitable) so as to prevent the breast falling over the baby's nose.

father to 'get to know their baby' thus helping to promote bonding and early attachment. Early suckling also releases the hormones prolactin and oxytocin which stimulate milk secretion and help the uterus to contract.

For the continued management of successful breast-feeding it is important for both the mother and the nurses to feel relaxed and at ease. Privacy must always be provided. The mother's position needs to be completely comfortable, and a low or easy chair with a suitable footstool can be of great assistance in achieving this. The mother should hold the baby comfortably in her arm but support from a pillow may be necessary to avoid fatigue. The baby must be allowed to play at the breast and nipple before starting to suck as this acts as an excellent stimulus for the milk flow. A little milk squeezed from the nipple may cause a baby who is slow to realize that he is expected to suck, to take the nipple into his mouth and start to feed. He should always be allowed to take the whole nipple and areola into his mouth or sucking may give the mother pain and cause sore nipples. The baby will also obtain less milk if he takes only the tip of the nipple into his mouth.

'On demand' rather than regular feeding allows frequent stimulation of the breast and nipple, reducing the time taken for milk production to become established. Mothers should not be expected to feed according to a rigid time-table.

Management of problems associated with breast-feeding

For mothers with poor lactation, the flow of milk can be stimulated by hot and cold bathing before starting to feed, by breast massage, by adequate support from a good brassière and by drinking of fluids. Mothers should be encouraged to express surplus milk after each feed, as this helps towards a better supply at the next feed.

Adequate washing and drying of the nipples will prevent them from cracking, a very painful condition for the mother and one which will interfere with successful breast-feeding.

The mother's general nutrition and state of health may need some attention as conditions such as anaemia or inadequate protein or kilojoule (Calorie) intake will produce poor lactation.

Complementary feeds. Complementary feeds are those offered after breast-feeds when these are insufficient. They are sometimes necessary as an interim measure until an adequate supply of breast milk is established. The baby may have been test-weighed to estimate the amount to be offered or he may be offered about two-thirds of his requirements and allowed to please himself.

A complementary feed should be either of boiled water or expressed breast milk. Substitute milk feeds should be avoided because they alter the intestinal bacterial flora and militate against successful breast-feeding. Complementary feeds should always be given by spoon as the technique of sucking from the breast is different to sucking from a bottle.

Supplementary feeds. Supplementary feeds are given to replace one or several entire breast-feeds per day. This may be done to rest the mother's nipples or because the mother is temporarily absent or indisposed. Again, the feed should be given by spoon in preference to a teat.

Artificial feeding

If breast-feeding is not possible, artificial milk feeds given to the baby should approximate to the composition of breast milk as nearly as is possible.

The success of infant feeding is assessed by the rate of growth. During the first few days of life the infant loses weight owing to passage of meconium and urine, the drying of the umbilical cord and the poor feed intake during this period. But, by the end of a fortnight, birthweight is regained. For the next 3 months the infant gains on average 170 g/week.

For the purpose of estimating the average feed requirements of the baby, it is necesary to know his expected weight, i.e. the weight he should be. It is useless to feed an underweight baby according to his actual weight as in this way he will never achieve his expected weight.

To calculate expected weight of infant

1. Take infant's birthweight.
2. After initial loss this should be regained by 10–14 days.
3. From 2 weeks to 3 months infant should gain 170 g/week.

Calorie* requirements in 24 hours

	Per kilogram of body weight in 24 hours
Pre-term infants (up to 2.5 kg)	130–150
Underweight infants	130–140
Normal infants	110–120

Fluid requirements in 24 hours

Premature infants (up to 1.4 kg)	250 ml
1.4–2.5 kg	220 ml
Infants over 2.5 kg	150–200 ml

Number of feeds in 24 hours

Up to 1.4 kg	2-hourly feeds × 10
Up to 2.5 kg	3-hourly feeds × 7
2.5–3 kg	4-hourly feeds × 6
3 kg upwards	4-hourly feeds × 5

Example to calculate feed for baby John

John's age	3 months
Birthweight	3.4 kg
170 g gain for (12 minus 2) weeks = 170 g × 10 =	1.7 kg
Expected weight is	5.1 kg

N.B. John's actual weight is 4.95 kg and so he is a little underweight.

(Remember that the aim is to feed to the expected weight for age.)

---

* Instead of measuring the energy value of foods in Calories there is a tendency to be correctly scientific and measure it in joules. Conversion is relatively easy if one remembers that approximately 4.2 joules = 1 calorie and 4.2 kilojoules = 1 kilocalorie (which is the large Calorie used in dietetics).

Calorie requirements for baby John
  5.1 kg × 115 ml = 586 Calories in 24 hours

Fluid requirements for baby John
  5.1 kg × 175 ml = 893 ml in 24 hours

Number of feeds in 24 hours
  4-hourly × 5 = 180 ml per feed
  Each feed contains 120 Calories
  30 ml contains 20 Calories
  (Calculations taken to the nearest whole number.)

Choice of artificial feeds

In the United Kingdom, artificial feeds intended to replace breast milk are manufactured as infant formulae. These may be powders or concentrated liquids which require reconstituting with water, or alternatively are sold already reconstituted in a 'ready-to-feed' form. Because breast milk is variable in composition, the composition of the artificial feed cannot be exactly the same as every sample of human breast milk, but it is usual for an artificial feed, which is reconstituted according to the manufacturer's instructions, to be comparable in respect to most nutrients with the average mature human milk from the healthy well-nourished mother.

Artificial infant formulae which are at present widely available in the United Kingdom may be classified into 3 categories.

Type 1
Cows' milk with added carbohydrate: Cow and Gate baby milk plus (added glucose); improved Ostermilk No. 2 (added maltodextrim).

Type 2
Skimmed cows' milk with added carbohydrate and mixed fats: Milumil (added maltodextrim and starch); SMA (added lactose).

Type 3
Skimmed cows' milk with demineralized whey and mixed fats: Cow and Gate premium; Osterfeed; SMA Gold Cap.
All 3 categories of artificial milk formula contain added minerals including iron, and added vitamins A, C and D. In some preparations certain trace elements may also have been added, e.g. copper, zinc and manganese.

The ready-to-feed concept
   Many hospitals have found the use of pre-packed feeds economical, much more convenient and labour saving as their use avoids the need for manufacturing bulk artificial feeds. The possible risk of infection is reduced also.
   Most hospitals using this method use one brand of feed only, to avoid confusion and to achieve economy in purchase. The pre-packed feed is available usually in disposable 120-ml bottles. Sterile, screw tight teat units are provided to fit the top of each bottle. Although these teat units can be disposed of after each feed, in practice it is more economical for each infant to keep his own teat unit. In between feeds the teat is placed in a sterilizing solution, e.g. hypochlorite or one of the other sterilizing preparations using potassium monopersulphate or sodium dichloro-isocyanurate, then rinsed in sterile water before use. The teat can then be replaced as necessary or disposed of when the infant is discharged home.
   The feed of one or two bottles, according to the infant's requirements, are taken to the cot-side along with a special bottle-opener. The bottle-top is removed and the teat unit screwed on to the bottle and the correct volume fed to the

1. Check the button is down on the cap. Warm the bottle of Ready-to-Feed by immersion in hot water (N.B. If desired Gold Cap SMA Ready-to-Feed need not be warmed and can be fed at room temperature.) Shake and remove the cap (You will hear the vacuum break).

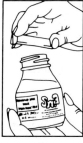

2. Strip the paper from bottom of teat unit.

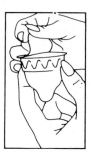

3. Screw teat unit on to bottle taking care to handle only the plastic ring. Do not touch the teat.

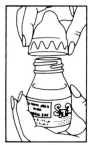

4. Remove plastic outer cover and check temperature, if necessary, by shaking a few drops on to the wrist.

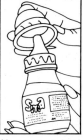

Preparation of Gold Cap SMA Ready-to-Feed could not be simpler. It only takes a few seconds and no measuring, mixing or sterilising is required. Bottles are graduated and it is easy to read-off the amount of feed baby has taken. Any Gold Cap SMA left over after feeding should be discarded, together with the glass bottle. There are two methods of dealing with the teat unit:

If a fully disposable system is employed, the complete unit is simply discarded along with the bottle and left-over feed.

If a part-disposable system is employed, then it is necessary to cleanse and sterilise the teat unit. Teats and rings may be re-sterilised by autoclaving or by immersion in an antiseptic (hypochlorite) solution. Cold sterilisation tends to prolong teat and ring life.

Fig. 7. How Gold Cap SMA Ready-to-Feed is administered.

infant as ordered. The teat unit is then removed, rinsed with cold water and returned to the ward kitchen where it can be disposed of appropriately. Sterile pre-packed feeds can be fed at room temperature or can be warmed up before the top is removed. Sterile pre-packed feeds may be kept for 3–6 months at room temperature.

Feeding the infant

Whenever possible the baby should be taken out of the cot for feeding, and held, comfortably wrapped, in the nurse's arms. He should have been changed recently and the hands should be washed again before feeding commences.

Feeding time should be used as an opportunity for cuddling and physical contact which play an important part in any infant's development but is particularly important for the baby deprived of his mother if she is unable to be with him.

The bottle should be held at a sufficiently steep angle to keep the teat constantly filled with milk and so prevent the baby from sucking in air. He should be allowed to bring up wind at least once during a feed, but babies who are sick often need to bring up wind very frequently often before starting as well as during the feed.

The teat should, if possible, be the one the baby is accustomed to, and the hole should be of a size which allows him to take his feed without much effort, and yet does not deliver the milk so quickly that he chokes. Inadequate holes can cause a baby to tire before completing the feed and so he refuses the last few millilitres, or swallows air by sucking hard without effect. Colic, vomiting and restlessness result.

When using an upright bottle it may be necessary to twist the bottle and teat while the baby is sucking, in order to allow air to enter and replace the milk, though many babies will let go from time to time and so prevent a vacuum forming, thus solving the problem for themselves.

Babies who are too eager or are underfed tend to gulp the first 60 ml or so, a habit which is likely to result in vomiting. A feed of 30 ml of boiled water before the milk formula is given, or an increase in the milk-feed are two ways of solving this problem. Failure to bring up wind, and excess crying due to hunger or discomfort between feeds may cause air swallowing with distension which may in turn cause vomiting.

A blocked nose can cause quite serious difficulty in feeding and can be one of the most commonly missed reasons for refusal of feeds. The nasal passages may be cleaned by inserting a wisp of cotton wool in the anterior nares, so inducing sneezing, alternatively nasal drops may be prescribed for a short time. Any baby with a blocked nose will take feeds more easily by spoon, as he is unable to breathe adequately with a teat in his mouth.

Bringing up wind

It is important to help the baby to bring up his wind, if unnecessary regurgitations, vomiting and colic are to be avoided. The baby should be sat on the nurse's lap, his head and body well supported, or alternatively laid over the nurse's shoulder and his back either rubbed or gently patted. This is comforting to the baby and appears to help in obtaining the desired effect. The principle is of course that of the air bubble which rises in a bottle. All babies swallow air when crying or feeding, and the nurse should not be satisfied until the baby has had at least one good eructation. Babies who cry a lot should be allowed to bring up wind before starting to feed.

Equipment

Bottles. There are many types of bottle obtainable but the most commonly used is the upright, heat resistant glass bottle. The upright type is easy to store and to handle, but it is not always easy to clean. The wider neck of the upright bottle has the advantage that it is easy to fill and much more easily cleaned.

Teats. It is often a good idea to experiment with teats to find the one to suit the particular infant's needs best. A strong rubber teat is good for babies who suck strongly and is obtainable in three sizes of hole: small, medium and large. The softer teat with airflow is helpful for babies with a poor sucking reflex. Long-lasting silicone teats are available that fit any sized neck bottle but these have the disadvantage of being expensive.

Sterilization

The sterilization of equipment can be carried out by boiling, autoclaving or immersion in a chemical solution, e.g. hypochlorite liquid according to the manufacturer's instructions.

The success of any of these methods is entirely dependent upon thorough cleanliness before sterilization in order to completely remove all traces of milk curd and fat.

Bottles will be easier to clean if each one is rinsed after use and filled with cold water. The use of hot water for this purpose will congeal the milk protein and make the bottle very difficult to clean; teats should also be rinsed immediately after use and some cold water squeezed through the holes.

Later the bottles can be washed using a soapless or detergent cleaner, hot water and a bottle brush and then sterilized. Teats should be rubbed inside and out with salt to remove any milk deposits, thoroughly rinsed in cold water before sterilizing.

If the hypochlorite method of sterilizing is used, it is important to remember that the solution must be changed every 24 hours.

Preparation of an individual feed

Thorough cleanliness is essential. After setting out the materials required, the nurse should again wash her hands.

The mixing instructions on the packet or formula container should be followed implicitly. Accuracy is essential.

To dilute infant formula made in the United Kingdom use:

1 level scoop of powder with each 30 ml (1 oz) measured volume of boiled water.

Scoops should be measured accurately and levelled with the edge of a knife.

Do not
Measure scoop by pressing against the inside of the packet or tin.
Compress milk powder in the scoop.
Add sugar or solids to the bottle.
Add or subtract an extra measure of powder.
Use a scoop measure made for one brand of milk powder with another.

Discharge home
When an artificially fed infant is being discharged home, always ensure the mother knows how to make up the feeds. If necessary demonstrate home method in the ward kitchen to the mother and always give written instructions before she leaves the ward. Ensure the mother has adequate supplies of infant formula at home prior to discharge.

Some feeding difficulties

Vomiting. There are some babies who vomit more readily than others and this must always be investigated as the small baby can very quickly lose essential water and minerals and become dehydrated.

When describing a vomit, the nurse should always state whether it was forcible or effortless, and when it occurred in relation to the feeds. She should describe the appearance of the vomit, the presence of curds, blood or mucus and the apparent stage of digestion.

There are very many causes for vomiting in infancy, some of which are directly related to feeding including: failure to bring up wind adequately, sucking from a teat with too small a hole, gulping a feed too quickly and finger sucking associated with air swallowing. Once pathological causes for vomiting have been excluded the nurse should advise the other how to remedy any other cause.

Regurgitation and posseting. This should not be confused with vomiting. In these babies a small amount of the feed is returned on bringing up wind or between feeds. It is rarely of importance, but is often a sign that a little too much feed is being offered.

Principles of weaning

The introduction of solid foods should be commenced somewhere between the ages of 4–6 months. Weaning is a gradual process which may take several weeks to achieve. This allows the infant time to adapt to new tastes, textures and a new method of feeding.

Gradually, the infant becomes less dependent on milk. By the age of 1 year, although milk is still an important food source, the infant will now be able to partake of a variety of other foods which provide good dietary sources of iron with differing tastes and textures.

Introducing solid foods

Additions to the diet should be tried 2–3 days before a further addition is tried, and if the baby obviously dislikes the taste after a few days then the addition should be omitted and tried again later.

Baby cereals mixed with milk are commonly the first

foods introduced. A rice-based (gluten-free) one should be chosen initially. The additions to the diet should be given with a spoon. As the amount of solid food increases, feed volume should be reduced to prevent obesity. Extra fluids such as water or fruit juice should be offered to quench the thirst.

A large choice of commercially prepared weaning foods is available, and although they are convenient they are also expensive. Home-cooked puréed foods are cheaper and nutritionally suitable, providing salt or salty gravy has been avoided. Sugar should be used sparingly as a sweetener. Because of the poor iron content of milk, iron-containing foods such as egg yolk, red meat and liver should be included in the diet. As the baby becomes accustomed to the mixed diet the times of the feeds can be altered to fit in with the household mealtimes if these are the most convenient for the mother.

Vitamins

Young infants who are breast-fed by a well-nourished mother already receive an adequate supply of vitamins. Infants artificially fed with an approved proprietary milk formula will also receive sufficient for their growth needs.

When mixed feeding is introduced, however, there is a risk that vitamin deficiency can occur. The DHSS report (1983) on Present Day Practice in Infant Feeding (HMSO) recommends that all infants from the age of one month should receive 5 drops daily of the 'Children's Vitamins Drops' available nationally through the Welfare Food Scheme. This should be continued until the infant is at least 2 years old or preferably 5 years old. The single dose of 5 drops contains approximately:

Vitamin A—200 μg
Vitamin C—20 μg
Vitamin D—7 μg

These vitamins for infants and young children are available to parents under the Welfare Food Scheme either free of charge or at reduced cost.

PLANNING FOR DISCHARGE HOME

This should begin early and involve all members of the caring team. The following is a basic check list to ensure that the parents are adequately prepared for the discharge home of their baby.

1. Environment. As the baby may have arrived earlier than expected, have the parents had time to obtain all the necessary essentials, e.g. clothing, nappies and cot? Are they aware of the need for the room temperature to be comfortably warm to protect their infant against hypothermia?

2. Infant feeding. If the baby is artificially fed, does the mother understand fully the making up of feeds? Does she have all the necessary utensils? Does she know of how/where to obtain further supplies of the milk formula? A written list of details is helpful for her to take home and refer to.

3. Equipment/supplies and drugs medication. Does the infant require any of these? Are the parents familiar with their use/reasons for these? Have adequate supplies been given to the parents until the next appointment? Do the parents appreciate the significance of ensuring that all drugs are kept within a locked cupboard?

4. Bathing. Is the mother confident and happy with this procedure? Has it needed modifying to fit in with her home conditions?

5. Has the mother been given an out-patient appointment for her infant? Provide her with written details of time, etc. Ensure that she is happy with the time and date provided. Are they convenient for her to keep?

6. The nurse should inform the health visitor before the discharge home, at least 48 hours beforehand. Do the parents know her name and that of the nearest child health clinic? Ensure that the health visitor receives a summary of the infant's nursing care whilst in hospital and any notes for future care.

Further reading

BATES, S. (1979) *Practical Paediatric Nursing*, 2nd edn. Oxford: Blackwell Scientific.

COCKBURN, F. & DRILLIEN. C. M. (1974) *Neonatal Medicine*. Oxford: Blackwell Scientific.

KELNAR, C. J. H. & HARVEY, D. (1981) *The Sick Newborn Baby*. London: Baillière Tindall.

RICKMAN, P. P. & JOHNSTON, J. H. (1978) *Neonatal Surgery*, 2nd edn. London: Butterworth.

VULLIAMY, D. G. (1977) *Newborn Child*, 4th edn. Edinburgh: Churchill Livingstone.

3 The infant at risk

The parents of infants who are born either before term, of low birthweight, or with abnormalities will need help in coping with this stressful situation. Inevitably, the shock of learning that their baby is small and immature or is suffering from a physical or mental handicap will be very great. Much time, sympathy and understanding is needed to help the parents come to terms with their situation. They will need to ask many questions from a variety of people. In hospital, the doctor and the senior nurse should be the ones to discuss the parents' problems with initially. Later, the paediatric liaison health visitor, medical social worker and others will support and counsel the parents.

Babies who have undergone a difficult birth, have suffered from an infection in the perinatal period, those with a history of genetic disorder, low birthweight infants, those with respiratory distress and other infants with an acute perinatal problem are amongst those who will need particularly careful observation and nursing care. This is best given in the Special Care Baby Units which provide neonatal intensive care by nurses and midwives especially trained and interested in this special branch of nursing. Prompt recognition treatment and specialized nursing care can be assured in this way together with the most modern equipment and technology.

Close liaison with the pediatric health visitor will not only ensure continuity in the care of these infants and their families but may also mean the detection of other problems which may present in the first few weeks of life. Certain tests are now carried out routinely within this early period, e.g. the Guthrie test to detect phenylketonuria, an inherited metabolic disorder.

ATTACHMENT OR MOTHER/INFANT BONDING

Klaus, Kennell and Trause define attachment 'as a unique emotional relationship between two people which is specific and endures through time'. This attachment has been shown to commence with delivery of the infant to the mother.

It is important for paediatric nurses to have insight and knowledge of this special relationship in order that they can promote the relationship despite the adverse situation of the infant requiring prolonged hospital care and treatment.

Physical contact

The mother should have the opportunity to hold her baby quietly, to fondle and to suckle the infant unless this is specifically excluded for any clinical reason. For the infant who has to be removed immediately from the delivery room the mother should, at the earliest opportunity, be given a polaroid or 'instant' photograph of her baby and allowed to visit her baby; fathers, too, should be included.

Participation in care

The opportunity for the mother to be involved in care is important for the development of attachment. The mother at first may feel a reluctance to do this, especially if her infant is pre-term, very low birthweight or obviously handicapped. The mother will be finding it difficult to adjust to her 'less than perfect child' when her expectations were for a perfect baby to take home soon after delivery.

The nurse will need to show the mother how to hold and fondle her baby in an environment which must seem very bewildering and strange.

The 'role model' of the nurse is particularly important. The nurse should show by her actions that she sees the child as an individual by using the child's first name and talking to it gently as she provides care. This will give the mother confidence and courage to take on the caring opportunities that the nurse is able to provide for the mother to do, e.g. changing a nappy even though the infant is in an incubator.

The nurse should take great care also to explain to the mother 'unit policies', e.g. hand washing protocols and why they are important to the well-being of her infant. Every effort should be made, too, to keep the mother informed of all developments and changes in her baby's condition.

Siblings and grandparents can also play an important role in visiting the unit and thus providing support for the parents.

A record should be kept of parental visiting and of their progress in caring for their infant. In this way, the possibility of any rejection can be foreseen early. When planning for discharge, it is helpful for the family health visitor to be provided with a summary of this information.

DEFINITIONS

Traditionally, infants under 2.5 kg (5½ lb) were called 'premature'. It is now recognized that weight alone is not sufficient for estimating gestational age or for planning nursing care. The infant at 'term' is one who is born after 37 weeks' gestation and before 42 weeks' gestation and weighing 2.5 kg or more.

Pre-term infants

These infants are small and of less than 37 weeks' gestation. Nursing care is directly related to the degree of immaturity.

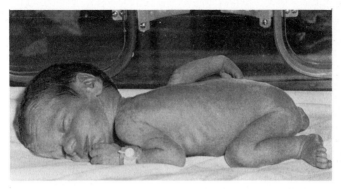

Fig. 8. The normal posture of the premature infant.

Low birthweight infants, or small-for-gestational-age infants

These infants are small due to poor intrauterine nutrition, often due to maternal health problems.

Characteristics of these small infants

1. Their heads appear large in comparison to the rest of the body.

2. They have a feeble cry, but often appear most alert.

3. Marked lack of subcutaneous tissue, dry loose skin with absence of skin creases.

4. Scalp hair is sparse, nails soft and external genitalia immature.

5. Irregular respiration.

Post-mature infants

These infants born after 42 weeks' gestation vary considerably in birthweight. Due to placental deterioration *in utero*, these babies often tolerate the stress of delivery poorly and may suffer from hypoxia, meconium aspiration and jaundice. The body appears thin and long due to wasting of subcutaneous fat. The nails are often long and the hair profuse.

The handicapped child

Infants born with handicapping conditions may be either pre-term, term or post-mature. The condition may not be apparent immediately at birth.

Congenital anatomical abnormalities

A list of the more common types is of interest.

The head. Microcephaly, hydrocephaly, oxycephaly, naevi, choanal atresia.

The eye. Buphthalmos, congenital cataract, strabismus, microphthalmia.

Ears. Absence of the pinna or meatus, congenital deafness, Bat ears.

Mouth. Cleft lip (hare lip), cleft palate, micrognathia (congenital smallness of the lower jaw).

Alimentary tract. Pyloric stenosis, oesophageal atresia, tracheo-oesophageal fistula, hiatus hernia, Hirschsprung's disease, imperforate anus, congenital obliteration of the bile duct, meconium ileus, rectovaginal fistula.

Bones. Osteogenesis imperfecta, spina bifida, achondroplasia, syndactyly, talipes, congenital dislocation of the hip joint, missing bones.

Thorax. Diaphragmatic hernia, congenital heart disease (with or without cyanosis).

Abdomen. Varieties of hernia, exomphalos.

Genito-urinary tract. Horse-shoe kidney, double ureters, hypospadias, epispadias, rectovaginal fistula, pseudo-hermaphroditism, hydrocele, undescended testicles, ectopia vesicae.

Central nervous system. Cystic spina bifida (meningocele, myelomeningocele), anencephaly, microcephaly, hydrocephaly and a variety of conditions which may be responsible for cerebral palsy.

THE NURSING ENVIRONMENT

Temperature

These infants all need to be protected against heat loss as they are vulnerable to hypothermia. This results in increased oxygen consumption and metabolic rate, loss of weight, lethargy and may result in death. The methods used to achieve and sustain a stable body temperature must depend upon the infant's age, maturity and size. Care should be taken to avoid increasing the infant's temperature rapidly as this places considerable stress on the infant's metabolic requirements.

The nursery temperature needs to be over 25°C for infants weighing about 2000 g and up to 30°C for those infants weighing less than 2000 g.

Radiant warmer

An overhead radiant warmer maintained by 'Servo Control' over an open base or cot provides the nursing staff with good access to the infant for care and observations.

Incubator

As an enclosed box-like environment, the incubator can be set at a particular environmental temperature or the infant can be attached to a temperature probe and the incubator maintained on 'Servo Control'. Oxygen and humidity can be delivered into the incubator at pre-set levels. Care needs to be taken that the incubator is not placed in direct sunlight to avoid creating the 'glasshouse' effect and thus increasing the ambient temperature. The infant is nursed naked but may wear a stockinette or knitted cap to prevent further radiant heat loss through the scalp.

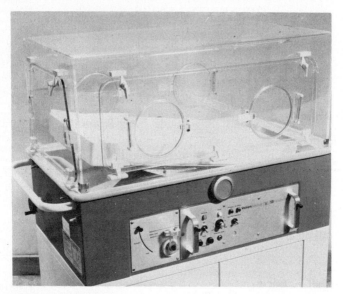

Fig. 9. An incubator.

Cot
Infants who are progressing and maintaining a stable temperature can be nursed clothed and in a cot or small crib.

Respiratory assistance—oxygen therapy
Oxygen is essential to the body for the production of energy. Oxygen therapy may be needed in the treatment of respiratory failure and to relieve hypoxia. Oxygen levels should be monitored frequently and regularly by blood gas analysis and transcutaneous oxygen measurements. Maintenance levels of administered oxygen should be ordered by the paediatrician according to clinical need and maturity of the infant.

Excessive oxygen therapy has been shown to have an adverse effect upon the retina of the eye producing 'retrolental fibroplasia' and in the lungs of immature infants, resulting in 'bronchopulmonary dysplasia'.

Oxygen may be administered through an incubator, oxygen hood, croupette, oxygen tent, or a paediatric face mask (see p. 156).

Mechanical ventilation

The decision to use mechanical ventilation for the infant will be made on the following criteria:

Cyanosis unrelieved by high oxygen levels.
Apnoea with depressed respiratory rate.
Blood oxygen levels below 50 mmHg in 100%.
P_{CO_2} between 60–70 mgHg in 100%.
pH below 7.2.

The nursing management considerations of an infant requiring mechanical ventilation are basically the same as for the older child, with the following exceptions. As the risk of infection is very great, due to the immature immunological systems of the 'infant at risk', sterile precautions should always be used for changing the ventilator tubing every 12–24 hours and suctioning of the airway.

N.B. Routine cultures should be taken daily after incubation.

Chest physiotherapy

Consultation with physiotherapist colleagues will be required in the presence of atelectasis and excessive mucous secretions. In some instances this treatment will be carried out by the nurse.

Chest physiotherapy should never be performed till 30–45 min after the last feed. Care should be taken not to exhaust the infant and vital signs should be monitored frequently. As 'cupped hands' are too large for the chest vibration in these small neonates, a vibrator or padded battery-operated toothbrush may be used most effectively.

NUTRITION

Adequate kilojoule (Calorie) intake is essential for optimal brain growth, to meet metabolic needs and to provide for normal growth development; the low birthweight infant requires at least 130 Calories/kg/24 h.

Breast-feeding

Every effort should be made to support and assist the mother to produce her own milk if she wishes to breast-feed, even though at this stage the baby may be too weak or sick to suck at her breast.

The midwife will instruct the mother in the use of either an electric or hand pump (these may be borrowed or hired at low cost from the Health Authority or voluntary organizations, e.g. National Childbirth Trust) or to express her milk manually.

It is important that the mother understands the need to express her milk regularly at 3–4-hourly intervals to avoid engorgement of her breasts. At first, the milk supply may be poor, but if the breasts have been regularly expressed the supply will increase once the infant begins sucking at the breast.

Ideally, the milk should be collected, labelled and delivered daily to the ward so that it can be given to her baby without being frozen. Plastic bottles or bags are better for collection as leucocytes in the milk adhere to glass surfaces.

Artificial feeding

There are many suitable artificial formulae available. The final choice must depend on the special needs of the infant, the mother's preference and unit policy.

Table 1. Methods of feeding

Route	Indications
Nasogastric Allow to flow in by gravity. Too rapid a feed may cause abdominal distension or regurgitation	Employed for infants unable to suck
Duodenal/jejunal Feed given by slow drip or continuous infusion. N.B. Gastric catheter may also be in-situ to reduce abdominal distension and check gastric aspirate	For infants requiring mechanical ventilation and for those who are very small or ill
Gastrostomy Feed given by gravity	Usually used postoperatively and for infants requiring prolonged artificial feeding
Bottle and teat/breast May be introduced initially to alternate with nasogastric feeding to avoid exhaustion of the infant	For the infant who is vigorous and able to suck well
Total parenteral nutrition An infusion to provide protein, carbohydrate and fats can be given either through a peripheral or central venous line	Most often used postoperatively or for those infants unable to feed orally for prolonged periods

GENERAL CARE

Observation

This is the most important tool of the nurse caring for the 'infant at risk'. Continued, intelligent observation of appearance, posture, activity and elimination will provide information for assessing progress and planning future care.

Cleanliness

The nature and frequency of bathing the infant would

depend upon unit policy and the particular condition of the infant. The napkin area is cleansed at each nappy change using hexachlorophane 3% or sterile water.

Eye care

These should be cleaned daily with a single cotton wool ball soaked in sterile warm water, then wiped dry. A separate swab should be used for each eye and each movement.

Nostril care

Leave untouched but if blocked with secretions, wipe external nares gently; this will often stimulate sneezing and clear the obstruction.

Cord care

See p. 25.

SUMMARY OF NURSING CARE

1. Carefully planned and minimal nursing intervention.
2. Control of oxygen administration.
3. Protection of infant against heat loss or excessive heat gain.
4. Correction of abnormal blood chemistry.
5. Careful, adequate feeding.
6. Maintenance of respiration possibly with mechanical assistance.
7. Prevention of infection.
8. Maintenance of parental and family links.

SOME NEONATAL PROBLEMS

Haemorrhagic disease of the newborn

Occasionally a baby may suddenly vomit blood or pass a melaena stool or blood-stained urine, or may be found to be bleeding from the nose, vagina or umbilicus. The bleeding occurs without warning and is most common from the third day onwards. The cause is lack of vitamin K, which in turn causes hypoprothrombinaemia and an abnormally long prothrombin time, usually only seen in breast-fed infants.

Treatment by giving vitamin K (1–2 mg by intramuscular injection) must not be delayed.

Occasionally a small vomit of altered blood or a melaena stool are caused by the baby swallowing blood as, for instance, during birth or from the mother's cracked nipple. It is for the doctor to decide and confirm the cause of any such signs of bleeding and the nurse must report them promptly and save the abnormal stool or vomit for inspection.

Haemolytic disease of the newborn
(rhesus incompatibility)

Neither Rh-positive or Rh-negative individuals normally have anti-Rh antibodies in their serum, but if a Rh-negative woman bears a Rh-positive child or fetus she may develop anti-Rh antibodies. With future pregnancies these antibodies can pass via the placenta into the fetal circulation causing the red cells to haemolize resulting in anaemia and jaundice of the newborn infant.

All Rh-negative mothers of Rh-positive babies are now given anti-D gamma-globulin within 36 hours of delivery to prevent rhesus incompatibility problems with future pregnancies.

However, if rhesus incompatibility does occur the principal manifestations are:

1. Stillbirth or death within a few hours, associated with hydrops fetalis.
2. Icterus gravis.
3. Congenital anaemia.

Newborn infants with anaemia and jaundice resulting from rhesus incompatibility must be treated as soon as possible after birth with an exchange transfusion.

Sclerema

Sclerema is associated with a thickening of the subcutaneous tissues, most noticeably in the back, buttocks and legs. The skin is cold and hard to touch. The exact cause is unknown, but implicated factors have been found to be:

Hypothermia.
Reduced peripheral circulation.
Staphylococcal or streptococcal infection.

Nursing management and treatment

This is planned to:

1. Monitor body temperature and gradually re-warm the infant.

2. Correct any metabolic problem, e.g. acidosis with intravenous therapy.

3. To provide for energy requirements and to avoid undue exertion of the infant by tube feeding, if possible with mother's own milk.

4. Combat infection. Commence antibiotics. Exchange transfusion is sometimes helpful by providing factors to aid the infant's own immunity system.

Respiratory distress syndrome

Affects mainly the pre-term infant, and is due to a deficiency of surfactant (an enzyme which lowers the surface tension of the alveoli). This leads to alveolar collapse, dilated alveolar ducts and pulmonary congestion. The blood supply to the kidneys and the gastrointestinal tract is impaired. Oedema is often marked. Respiratory acidosis is present with consequent electrolyte disturbances.

The syndrome may occur immediately after birth or within a few hours of delivery. Most commonly affects males, born by caesarian section and in those with a sibling history of respiratory distress. Maternal diabetes and rhesus isoimmunization increases the incidence.

Nursing management and treatment

This is planned to:

1a. Decrease energy requirements and therefore oxygen consumption. Place infant under radiant warmer or in an incubator with less than 30% oxygen. Blood gases and pH monitored frequently. Mechanical ventilation may become necessary if respiratory failure occurs.

1b. Nursing intervention reduced to a minimum to decrease stress.

Monitor continuously: heart rate; respiratory rate; transcutaneous P_{O_2}; temperature.

Monitor frequently: Dextrostix for hypoglycaemia; blood pressure.

Measure urine output and specific gravity.

2. Meet fluid and nutrition requirements initially by feeding intravenously with 5% dextrose. As improvement occurs nasogastric feeding is slowly introduced.

3. Antibiotics may be ordered either to treat infection or as prophylaxis.

Jaundice

This is a yellow discolouration of the skin due to the accumulation of bilirubin. Bilirubin is the product of the breakdown of the 'haem' portion of haemoglobin, and exists in two forms, albumin-bound and free. Bilirubin is normally excreted in the bile into the duodenum.

Physiological jaundice

Usually first noticed about 24 hours after birth, reaching

a peak about 4–5 days later. This condition results from the increased breakdown of red blood cells and immature liver function; usually more severe in pre-term infants. Serum bilirubin levels may be increased by dehydration and poor feeding, and also occurs in some breast-fed infants.

Treatment. Close monitoring of serum bilirubin levels. No active treatment indicated unless bilirubin levels rise above 140–170 mmol/litre for infants weighing 2000–2500 g, when phototherapy may be indicated.

Kernicterus

Kernicterus is the development of brain damage secondary to the deposition of bilirubin in the brain cells.

Initially the infant may appear yellow and lethargic, with poor sucking and a high pitched cry. Hypotonia or hypertonia with downward rolling of the eyes may be present. Apnoea and fits may also occur. Without recognition and treatment, permanent spasticity with mental handicap will result.

Treatment. Exchange transfusion after initial infusion of albumin 1 g/kg.

Necrotizing enterocolitis

Disease of the bowel resulting in patches of necrotic mucosa and intramural gas, leading to severe abdominal distension, bleeding in the bowel and collapse. Precise cause unknown, but associated factors include prematurity, asphyxia, hypothermia, hypoglycaemia, and acidosis.

Onset is sudden, between 1–14 days after birth, but most commonly between 4–7 days.

Nursing management and treatment

Care and treatment depend upon the stage of disease when a diagnosis is made.

Early diagnosis
   Gastric decompression with nasogastric tube.
   Total parenteral nutrition.
   Broad spectrum antibiotics after specimen cultures have
been made of blood, gastric aspirate and faeces.

Late diagnosis
   As above, but proceeds to surgery for resection of any
perforated, gangrenous bowel.

N.B. Prevention. Be alert to signs, note and report in
vulnerable infants:

   Increased amounts of gastric aspirate.
   Abdominal distension—measure every 2–4 hours.
Report any increase over 1 cm.
   Test stools for occult blood.

Ophthalmia neonatorum

Any prudent discharge from the eye within 21 days of birth
is notifiable, irrespective of the cause. The commonest
causative organisms are staphylococcus and gonococcus.
   Ophthalmia neonatorum once accounted for a high proportion of blindness in children, but nowadays owing to
adequate prophylaxis and treatment with antibiotics, eye
infections rarely have serious consequences. Symptoms
vary from slight oedema of the eyelids, inability to open the
eyes and presence of frank pus, to changes in the eye itself.

Nursing management and treatment

   Infants with 'sticky eyes' should be nursed with strict
precautions against spread of infection and should be carefully isolated from other babies with a special nurse attending them.
   Appropriate antibiotic ophthalmic ointment is prescribed. If drops are ordered the following routine may be
followed: one drop is instilled every minute for the first

½-hour, then every 5 min until all discharge disappears (usually a further hour) then ½-hourly until the swelling subsides (usually another 8–12 hours) then every hour for 12 hours, and every 2 hours for another 24 hours after that. This treatment is modified according to the wishes of the doctor. If one eye only is affected, the infant should be nursed on the affected side to prevent discharge from running over the bridge of the nose into the healthy eye. The baby's arms must be effectively restrained to prevent him from touching his eyes and so spreading the infection.

If the infection persists blockage of the lacrimal duct should be suspected.

Naevi or birth marks

Naevi (singular: naevus) consist of a localized cluster of dilated blood vessels. There are various types of naevi, some of which are present at birth, others appear some months later. Of the different types most disappear spontaneously but others persist. Some naevi are very extensive and may disfigure an entire side of the face or cause enlargement of the tongue associated with difficulty of speech, eating and breathing.

CHILD ABUSE/NON-ACCIDENTAL INJURY

It has been increasingly recognized over recent years that some young children suffer repeated injury at the hands of their parents. The nurse should always remember that the reasons are very complex. Young parents in an overcrowded home and short of money may feel it to be the last straw when faced with a constantly crying child and give vent to their feelings. The nurse should never judge but attempt to understand and support the parents whilst at the same time protecting the child.

Many such children appear well cared for and loved, and

the assault by one or other of the parents appears due to momentary loss of control. Other children may be present with profound physical and emotional neglect. Often the bruising and haematoma are obvious but occasionally rib and other fractures are detected by radiographs, taken for other reasons; and the parents may give no history of previous injury.

If the doctor or nurse has any doubt about the cause of the injury the following recommendations were made by the British Paediatric Association in 1966.

1. The child is admitted to hospital for appropriate treatment.

2. A detailed medical history is obtained with all the possible information about the family from the family doctor and the health visitor.

3. When all information is obtained the paediatrician should have a personal interview with the parents. If the evidence of inflicted injury is scanty, on discharge of the child the medical social worker should liaise closely with the family doctor and health visitor in order that supervision and social support can be given to the family to prevent further episodes and family breakdown. If the evidence is more definite the consultant should advise the parents that he is informing the Director of Social Services and that meanwhile the child will be kept in hospital. If the parents insist on taking the child home the paediatrician will explain that he will inform the police in order that a warrant can be obtained from a justice of the peace to ensure that the child is kept in hospital or other 'safe place'.

This last action needs only to be resorted to in a minority of cases. Most consultants agree that it is best through the use of the psychiatric services and social agencies to concentrate on family rehabilitation and avoidance of further child abuse.

PAEDIATRIC PROCEDURES

Intravenous infusions

Stab
> Dressing pack.
> Disposable syringes.
> Suitable giving set and cannulae.
> Skin cleansing lotion.
> Infusion fluid (to be checked with prescription).
> Adhesive plaster, bandage and scissors.
> Protection for bed and patient's clothing.
> Padded and protected splint of suitable size.

Have available:
> Charts as necessary.
> Infusion stand.
> Restrainers or mitts as required.

Cut down
> Cut down pack.
> Sterile disposable gloves.
> Ampoule local anaesthetic.
> Intravenous giving set.
> Skin cleansing lotion.
> Infusion fluid (to be checked with prescription).
> Adhesive plaster, bandage and scissors.
> Protection for bed and patient's clothing.
> Padded and protected splint of suitable size.
> Charts as necessary.
> Infusion stand.
> Equipment for shaving head if necessary.
> Restrainers or mitts as required.

General nursing responsibilities

1. Prepare equipment. Check intravenous fluid with the doctor and prepare infusion.

2. Ensure parents understand the need for the infusion. Explain the procedure to a child old enough in a language he understands. Hold and comfort the child.

3. The veins most commonly used with young children are the internal saphenous and the antecubital veins, but with infants the superficial scalp veins or the veins on the back of the hand are often very satisfactory.

4. Once infusion is established check the child at regular intervals for:

Any leakage from infusion site.

Any swelling of infusion site.

Rate of flow against ordered intravenous regime.

N.B. The serial number of the intravenous fluid should be recorded on the patient's fluid chart.

Blood transfusions

The main indications for a blood transfusion to a child are:

To restore circulating volume, e.g. after haemorrhage.

To provide blood components which may be deficient in the child, e.g. platelets.

If blood is to be given, it will have to be cross-matched and grouped in the laboratory, but the doctor and nurse should check the label against the patient's record sheet. The amounts to be given in a specified time will be ordered by the doctor but will rarely exceed 10–15 ml per 600 g of body weight.

Equipment required is the same as for intravenous infusions.

Scalp vein infusion

For a scalp vein infusion, the infant's head is shaved over the parietal bone and an assistant holds the head securely. Once the needle is in position, it may be secured by strapping or by plaster of Paris approximately 7.5 cm (3 in.) in width (Fig. 10).

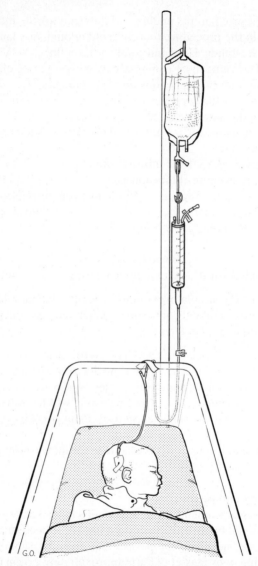

Fig. 10. Infant receiving intravenous therapy. (Note paediatric giving set.)

Table 2. Blood transfusions

Specific observations	Rationale
Immediately flow starts:	*For incompatibility reactions*
Record ¼-hourly pulse and hourly temperature	i.e. Rising pulse rate
	Sudden elevation of temperature (normal—97° F)
Observe colour and feel of skin and any respiratory distress	Twitching to convulsions
	Skin of face flushed
	May shiver
Estimate urinary output and concentration	Urinary output diminished
Throughout transfusion continue to:	*For allergic reaction to blood*
Record ¼-hourly pulse (rate/volume)	i.e. Appearance of shocked state
Observe respirations, colour and feel of skin and general appearance of infant	Respirations fluttering (very shallow and rapid)
	Where history in family (asthma, eczema or hay fever)
As for all infusions:	*To avoid overloading (also i.v.)*
Hourly recordings on i.v. chart	of circulation with possible heart failure or pulmonary oedema
Rate of flow—drops per min	
Amount given in that hour (1 drop = approx. 1/20th millilitre)	Maximum rate of intake 1 ml/lb/h
Frequently listen for bubbly sounds on respiration	
Note any cough or dyspnoea	
Any engorgement of neck veins	
Maintenance of rate of flow	*Difficulty of flow (also i.v.)*
If slowing down:	Rate ordered frequently very slow
Apply warmth to limb	
Check and adjust temperature of room	Also muscles around vein liable to go into spasm
Check splint and entry site of infusion	Easy to occlude circulation in newborn

Splinting for intravenous therapy

When a limb is used adequate splinting is essential and this is a highly skilled procedure, as immobility must be achieved without compressing important blood vessels. The splint should be well padded and covered in order to make it waterproof. For an infant, the splint need be only about 7.5 cm (3 in.) wide but the length should be sufficient to allow for it to support a loop of tubing. This takes the weight off the tubing and makes it possible to adjust the position of the needle in the vein by suitable padding. This method also minimizes the vibrations caused by restlessness or movement of the bottle which in turn helps to cut down inflammation within the vein. If the internal saphenous vein is used, the splint should reach from the fold of the buttock to about 25 cm (10 in.) beyond the toes or if a vein in the arm is used, from the head of the humerus to about 25 cm (10 in.) beyond the fingers. The foot and ankle are rotated externally and immobilized on the splint by lengths of 2.5 cm (1 in.) adhesive strapping passing across the heel just below the knee. In this way pressure on important blood vessels is avoided. If the antecubital vein is used, the arm is rotated externally and three lengths of strapping applied; one across the palm of the hand, one just below the antecubital fossa and the third high up on the arm and across the bony prominence of the shoulder. In either case a firm bandage and cotton wool are applied to give added immobility, but a space of about 5–7.5 cm (2 to 3 in.) is left uncovered so that the condition of the limb can be watched. A pad of foam sponge can be used to prevent foot-drop or an over-extension of the elbow. The splint should be firmly tied to the bed to ensure immobility.

Good splinting is essential, not only for the successful running of the intravenous drip infusion, but also because it enables the nursing staff to move the patient up and down the cot or to lift him out for feeding or weighing. In order to make this possible an extra length of sterile tubing should

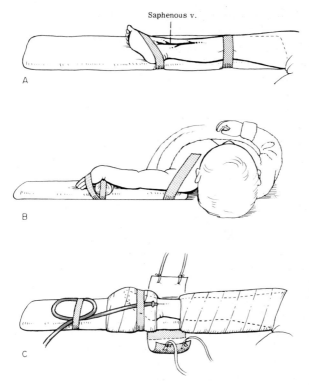

Saphenous v.

A

B

C

Fig. 11. (A) Correct splinting of leg for intravenous therapy. Note that any strapping used must be taken over a bony prominence to prevent constriction of blood vessels. (B) Correct splinting of arm for intravenous therapy into a vein of the dorsum of the hand. Note roll of foam sponge to prevent wrist drop. (C) A space is left between bandages for convenient and frequent inspection. The tubing is stabilized on the extra length of splint. This minimizes the movement and vibration and reduces risk of thrombosis or spasm of the vein.

always be attached to the adult giving set. Moving the patient at regular intervals is one way of preventing hypostatic pneumonia.

Care should be taken to see that the limb and splint are

not twisted and that neither groin nor tubing are kinked or constricted. It is a good plan to have a bed cradle over the limb, to facilitate inspection and to support the weight of the bedclothes.

Replacement transfusion
Dressing pack.
Disposable syringes.
Umbilical catheters of assorted sizes.
Skin cleansing lotion.
Sterile disposable exchange transfusion set containing instruments, stopcock with extension tubing and extra tubing.
Have available:
Charts as necessary.
Monitoring equipment.
Resuscitative equipment.
Laboratory forms and specimen bottles.
Fresh donor blood.
10% calcium gluconate.
50% glucose solution.
Sodium bicarbonate.
Sterile gown and gloves for the paediatrician.

Indications for replacement transfusion
Hyperbilirubinaemia.
Anaemia in rhesus incompatibility.
Polycythaemia—partial exchange with saline or plasma.
Severe sepsis.

Dangers
Air embolism, thrombosis, sepsis, acidosis, hypo-glycaemia, hypocalcaemia, bleeding, heart failure and nec-rotizing enterocolitis.

Nurse's responsibilities

1. Make sure the paediatrician has discussed the procedure with the parents and obtained their consent.

2. Ensure that the environmental temperature is sufficient to maintain the infant's body temperature.

3. Attach the infant to a cardiac monitor to record immediately any apnoea or bradycardia, if noted the procedure should be halted until condition stabilizes.

4. Check temperature, apex beat and respiration.

5. Aspirate stomach. Urine-collecting bag may be applied.

6. Secure the baby comfortably.

7. Check the blood with the paediatrician and record the serial number on the appropriate chart.

8. Note time of commencement and time of withdrawal and replacement of the blood. It should take approximately 1 min to remove and replace 10 ml of blood.

9. Check Dextrostix before commencement of procedure, half-way through procedure, and at the end of the exchange transfusion.

10. Make frequent recordings of heart rate, respiratory rate and pattern, also note the infant's colour.

11. At completion of the exchange transfusion closely observe the infant.

Check temperature, apex beat and respirations immediately and then at frequent intervals for at least 4 hours post-exchange transfusion. Observe the umbilicus for any bleeding.

Further reading

CROSS, V. M. (1975) *The Pretend Baby*. London: Churchill Livingstone.

NELIGEN, G. A., KOLVIN, I., SCOTT, D. McL. & GARSIDE, K. (1976) *Born too Soon and Born too Small*. London: Spac International Medical.

YOUNG, D. & WELLER, B. F. (1979) *Baby Surgery*. London: Harvey, Miller & Medcalf.

4 The needs of the sick child

Parents will need help in coping with the stressful situation of seeing their child sick or suffering pain. They may also be unfamiliar with hospital routine and even simple procedures they see carried out may, to them, seem traumatic or repulsive. It is also not easy for a mother, used to being in full charge of her child, to share this care and her authority with that of a nurse who to both of them is a stranger and who may, inadvertently, make the mother feel inadequate or embarrassed in the hospital surrounding. Fear of the outcome of an operation may change the parents' manner temporarily. They may withdraw or alternatively become very demanding. On the other hand, nurses may feel observed and criticized by experienced mothers and either avoid them and their children, or become officious and aggressive.

All these emotions add greatly to the stresses in a children's ward but if understood, make paediatric nursing all the more challenging and interesting.

Nurses dealing with children for the first time may well be puzzled by the problems arising from their behaviour. They will understand them far better if they consider them in relation to the child's family and social background. Children, in the same way as adults, are the product of their country, their district, their educational and social environment, and their daily pursuits and contacts; but what applies to the adult applies to children in a far greater degree. The younger the child, the more dependent he will be on his mother or his mother substitute. It is important to realize that in some families the grandmother means as much to the young child as his mother, and that she often looks after him during the mother's absence at work. This should never be forgotten when visiting is considered. In addition, the pre-school child is defenceless and immature both in body and mind. He cannot express himself clearly. He has not yet learned to be adaptable and to make easy social contacts, and he misses his usual routine, his diet, familiar streets and familiar faces, occasionally beyond endurance. His emotional development is still immature and he lives in the present, incapable of understanding a tomorrow. He has a lively imagination and readily inter-prets what he sees and hears into frightening fantasies. He is very sensitive to the tone of people's voices, to their gestures and to the expressions on their faces and may read fearful and alarming things into them. Doctors and nurses should always bear this in mind when talking about a child in a ward or outpatient department.

THE NURSING PROCESS AND SICK CHILDREN

The Nursing Process is essentially a problem-solving approach to the provision of nursing care. Duberly, a paediatric nurse, has written 'Nursing care is also influ-enced by the dependence of the patient upon others for his continuing care.' The Nursing Process therefore has a particular relevance to paediatric nursing as it allows for the recognition and integration of the child's dependence, developmental needs and those of his family unit.

The framework of the Nursing Process is classified in 4 stages:

1. Assessment
2. Planning
3. Implementation
4. Evaluation

These all overlap to some extent as the provision of nursing care is based on logical understanding and cannot be segmented into different zones.

Assessment

Essentially this is the stage of collecting information about the sick child which will allow the nurse, by identifying the child's problems, to make a nursing diagnosis. Then to be able to construct a nursing care plan which will meet identified goals and objectives of nursing care. This collection of information can be obtained by interview using a nursing assessment checklist.

The type used would depend on the age and development of the child, and the interview will often need to involve both child and mother/father/or other care giver. Account should be made for the child's own language and expression, e.g. his normal words for wanting to urinate. Equally, the assessment/interview should allow for the child's own interests/habits, if they effect his health, to be taken into account, e.g. is this 11-year-old asthmatic child smoking cigarettes?

Planning

Using the assessment information is the cornerstone for planning paediatric nursing care. Problems need to be identified and realistic goals set for the solution of the problems. The care plan can then relate the nursing actions to meet the identified goals.

Implementation

This is the giving of nursing care, taking into account all

the factors which influence the child's care. The ability of the mother/father to be resident and participating in the care is an important factor here. Example:

> Instruction of the resident parent in the collection and measurement of urine for a 24-hour sample for a 4-year-old with a suspected inborn error of metabolism is obviously important. The parent will know and be able to interpret their child's behaviour when he wishes to micturate, but will need to know the importance of accurate collection, and the use of the correct laboratory bottle and appropriate utensils. If for some reason the parent is not resident the nurse will need to implement a care plan that allows for an assigned nurse, using the assessment as the basis, to be in a position to know that when the child is restless and crossing her legs whilst deep in play, she wants to micturate, even if the pot had been emptied 10 min previously.

Evaluation

The evaluation or assessment of change can sometimes be obvious, but may also be most difficult when it is subtle and intangible. The assessment of change in the child's state or environment will often indicate a modification of the original care plans which will take into account that change. The frequency of that evaluation of the nursing care plan will vary, e.g. the low birthweight infant in a neonatal intensive care unit will need more frequent assessment than a 12-year-old on skeletal traction for a fractured femur.

Finally, apart from the value of the evaluation of the nursing care plans to the individual child, there are wider implications for the nurse which allow her to provide care to the child and his family in a unique and positive way, and by her evaluations to learn from past care plans which will influence the improved provision to others.

Table 3. Example of a nursing care plan

Victoria Fisher   Age   4 years

Date & code no.	Nursing problem	Objective	Nursing action & its rationale	Signature	Date disc.
3/8/83	Hot, flushed & pyrexial (temp. 38.8°C)	To relieve fever and promote comfort	Cool bathing and frequent changes of clothing Frequent cool drinks Monitor temperature 4-hourly		
	Runny sore nose	To promote healing of skin around nose	Apply zinc oxide cream to skin Provide soft paper tissues for nose blowing		
	Mucosy cough	To encourage expectoration to clear chest	Continue with tipping & tapping as agreed with physiotherapist		

4/8/83	Anorexic and lethargic	To promote appetite and return of energy	Provide small helpings of favourite foods—tomato soup
			        baked beans/chips
			        egg custard/ice cream
			Offer nourishing drinks—favourites include: hot chocolate
			        tea with sugar
			Encourage play activities which will stimulate and encourage social interaction, e.g. puppet play, cooking, collage making		

The hospital stay

The hospital experience may be deeply disturbing to children. To many of them being put to bed in the daytime implies punishment. This should be considered, particularly with children admitted from a waiting list or merely for investigations. They do not feel ill and to put them to bed on admission can only add insult to injury and serves no useful purpose. Some children share a bed at home and few are used to cot sides after the age of 2 to 3 years. To sleep alone in a high, white bed, surrounded by bars can in itself be a disturbing experience.

Nurses' uniform

The newly admitted child may never have seen people dressed in nurses' uniform and to some, hospital doctors and nurses have in the past been used as threats. It frequently happens that children are drawn to the ward cleaners, presumably because they wear less unfamiliar clothes and, in the case of a local hospital, talk the dialect to which the child is used.

As part of a policy to create a more attractive, less clinical environment on some paediatric wards the nurse is allowed to wear either a colourful attractive tabard or apron over her uniform, and in some places even to remove her traditional white cap. Other wards have abandoned uniform altogether.

Routine

Children are very dependent on a familiar routine, and no other person can imitate precisely the way in which the mother would set about the daily toilet or the dressing and undressing routine. This may lead to distress as well as protest. Children are readily labelled as having food fads. But here again, the child is used to certain foods, cooked and served in the way favoured by his mother at home.

Family menus are very repetitive and only rarely will hospital diet be anything like the meals to which the child has been used.

Using a pot may be a worrying experience to a child who at home is used to going to the lavatory but necessary for collection of urine and stool specimens. Occasionally children fail to use the pot when given one, only to wet or soil themselves a few moments after it has been taken away. This should be treated with understanding. It is often helpful to place the pot on a piece of macintosh on the floor where it is easier to balance than in bed, and where the child may feel more secure. To balance the pot in bed requires some skill and the child will inevitably tighten up his muscles including those of the bladder and anal sphincters. For that reason the child may be unable to use the pot but as soon as he comes off it and is able to relax, he wets and soils himself.

Visiting

Unrestricted visiting can make separation of mother and child more bearable and nurses should actively encourage parents to make full use of the facilities offered. Some parents are reluctant to visit because they think their child will cry when they have to leave. The nurse can explain to them that this is only to be expected, and that it is quite natural and far less harmful for the child that he should cry and be comforted than to feel abandoned because the parents do not visit.

Unrestricted visiting means that parents may be there at any time, and allows parents to be there at times when the child particularly needs them, e.g. at bedtime. It also means that the non-resident parent can choose to stay all day or to pop in and out according to their family needs.

Contact with home

Occasionally children cannot be visited, perhaps because they have come from a considerable distance. Arrangements should be made to keep up contact with home in every possible way. Examples of this are: daily postcards or parcels from home; telephone calls between mother and child; photographs of members of the family to be kept on the child's locker; school and evening prayers. Any such link with home will make the stay in hospital less traumatic.

Play

Play is a fundamental part of every child's inheritance through which he develops physically, emotionally and intellectually. It is through play that the child explores his environment, communicates and learns; there is no dividing line between work and play. Toys are the tools of play. Throughout childhood the child plays, at first through contact with his mother, then on his own and later with other children of his own age. With play, the child expresses his feelings and fantasies and thereby learns to cope with the reality of everyday life. Play has these same values for the sick child and the need increases with being in hospital away from his home and family. During illness the child regresses, becoming emotionally a little younger than his normal self, only able to concentrate for short periods and will play happily with easier toys than usual.

Often parents will ask for some guidance about suitable toys to buy as gifts. The nurse can remind them of their 'odds and ends' at home, the button box, the box of old keys, magazines, the rag bag, all of which will provide a link with home and are of occupational value. Other ideas that are inexpensive include, providing a special companion for the sick child with a hand puppet or rag doll, which not only provides friendship but enables the child to use the toy in dramatizing his situation. Toys that are too complicated or too involved should be avoided. Instead there should be things provided for the child to do, as well as visual stimulation, e.g. mobiles to hang on extension frames, snowstorm pictures or a felt board and scraps to make adjustable pictures. Children also need facilities for play apart from toys, e.g. a firm surface such as a bed table or tray, a 'play wall' for pinning up pictures, 'pop star' posters or drawings. Play containers for holding a child's precious toys may be a basket, box or bag, and for some children 'play arms' are useful, such as the aids used by the elderly to pick up objects from the floor or bed. Mirrors can be used to reflect activities in the ward and elastic bands to project paper messages or pellets to companions. If the ward has a play area the child should always be taken there, providing that his condition allows it, for set periods each day.

This play area should be sacrosanct and never used for treatments, medicines or medical examinations. An increasing number of children's units now have playgroups with playleaders as part of the ward team. Hospital play needs these specialists who are trained to provide suitable equipment and expertise for all ages of child confined to bed, wheelchair, or up and about, with a wide range of disabilities. The nurse needs to work closely with the playleader who should receive regular ward reports of each child's progress in order to ensure that individual needs are met. For those working in wards where there is not a playleader, the nurse should attempt to provide as much organized play as possible, involving parents and volunteers. The following guidelines will provide a general framework for the nurse to use:

1. Supply materials which stimulate play and allow expression.

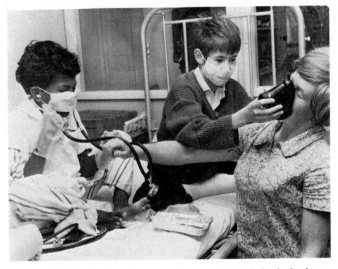

Fig. 12. Children playing at 'doctors and nurses' with their playleader as the patient, using old hospital equipment.

2. Playtime should be given priority in the ward routine and should be without interruption.

3. Allow the child to play at his own pace.

4. Play for and with the child who cannot play for himself.

5. Relate play to knowledge of each child's development.

The equipment provided should include simple creative craft materials, puppets, books, building-bricks, both board and card games as well as facilities for playing with sand, water, clay or dough. Children in hospital enjoy playing with ordinary household items and also hospital equipment such as stethoscopes, syringes (without needles), bandages and tubing, which allow them to act out their feelings about hospitalization. Wearing nurse's caps and face masks in bed as well as other dressing-up gear can be great fun for the child as well as being therapeutic, as an ill child who is happily occupied is likely to get well far more quickly than one who is not.

Giving medicines

The medicine round in a children's ward rarely presents much difficulty as children follow each other's example and the willingness of one readily infects the others. The key-note should always be a matter-of-fact attitude on the part of the nurse giving the medicine. To approach a child with an attitude of apology and a look of disgust, coupled with elaborate promises that it will not taste bad, is likely to court disaster. The child will feel that he is, as it were, expected to dislike the taste and to make a fuss. It is far better to carry on an ordinary conversation and so take the child's mind off the subject.

Medicines for children should be camouflaged to make them palatable. This is often done in the dispensary where brightly coloured syrups of various kinds are available. Medicines are usually taken better in solution than in tablet form. Both should be placed as far back on the tongue as possible and followed by a pleasant drink or a sweet chosen by the child himself from the ward sweet tin. Sometimes it is necessary to mix a drug with a drink or some semi-solid food such as a mashed banana or jam, but even if this is done, the child should be told that the medicine is there. In these cases it is important that the food chosen is not an essential one, in case the child becomes permanently suspicious of its taste. This applies, for instance, to milk, orange juice, mince and custard. Pre-operative drugs are often bitter. If they have to be camouflaged, syrup or honey are best, as they are quickly digested and the danger of vomiting and inhalation during anaesthesia does not arise.

Some children cooperate best if they are allowed to take the medicine from a coloured spoon, through a straw or polythene tube or from a doll's tea set. The nurse should be adaptable and use her imagination to the full. The trouble taken will be richly repaid. Drugs and medicines are best given at times not closely related to meals in case the child should vomit the feed or meal with the drug.

On the occasions where there is difficulty, it is sometimes best to take the child out of his cot and sit him on the nurse's knee safely wrapped in a small blanket. She may have to shape his mouth with one hand and pour the medicine in, but it should be remembered that this method is not without danger as a screaming, struggling child may well inhale some of the medicine thus forced into his mouth. Some medicines are best given by placing the spoon at the back of the tongue and letting the medicine go down by gravity. It is, as a rule, better to leave the child for a while and to return again later when his mood may have changed and he may be more cooperative. At all times, care must be taken to see that the whole dose is taken and that none is spat out or allowed to run down the chin or bib. Certain drugs are best followed by a small drink of water.

The effect of the drug given should be watched and recorded carefully and signs of intolerance reported at once. Punctuality in the giving is essential, as in many cases the efficacy depends on the concentration reached in the blood and a certain level may have to be maintained throughout the 24 hours. Children also get used to a certain routine and cooperate more readily if the medicine times follow a familiar pattern.

Dosage of drugs. Children's tolerance of drugs differs from that of adults; large dosages are often well tolerated. The dosage of drugs is often based on the child's body weight.

Accurate weight charts and the checking of weights by a qualified nurse are consequently important.

Body weight formula for calculating paediatric drug dosage:

$$\frac{\text{Child's weight (kg)}}{70} \times \text{adult dose}$$

$$\frac{\text{Child's weight (lb)}}{150} \times \text{adult dose}$$

Children require a higher dose per kilogram body weight than adults, since they have a higher metabolic rate.

Body surface measurements are more accurate for calculation of paediatric doses.

The following formulae are used to estimate the paediatric dosage based on the child's body surface area.

1. $\dfrac{\text{Surface area of child (m}^2)}{1.75} \times \text{adult dose} = \text{child dose}$

2. $\dfrac{\text{Surface area of child}}{\text{Surface area of adult}} \times \text{dose of adult}$

   $= \text{approximate child dose}$

3. Surface area $(m^2) \times \text{dose/m}^2 = \text{approximate child dose}$

Resuscitation

The nurse working in a children's ward must be able to deal effectively with cardiac arrest. Not only may the heart have stopped suddenly, but breathing may also have ceased. A pulse may be absent and the pupils may be dilated.

In this situation one nurse will usually begin resuscitation of the child, while another calls for medical aid and fetches the resuscitation box or trolley. As the emergency procedure varies from hospital to hospital, all nurses must acquaint themselves with the set procedure within their own hospital. As with the adult patient, success depends on team work. The aim of emergency resuscitation is the restoration of an effective circulation of oxygenated blood by means of artificial ventilation and external cardiac massage. Speed is essential to ensure survival of the brain cells which can only survive undamaged without oxygen for approximately 3 min.

Artificial ventilation. The first essential is to establish and maintain a clear airway by hyperextending the head and pulling the chin forward, as obstruction will prevent adequate ventilation. A quick check should be made that vomit is not present in the mouth, by placing a finger in the mouth. If the child has vomited, the vomit should be allowed to drain away by tilting the head and chest downwards.

Mouth to mouth breathing must be started if a rebreathing bag (e.g. Ambu type) is not available. The nurse using her own lungs as a positive respirator, can ventilate the patient's lungs. If the child is small enough the nurse places her mouth over both the patient's nose and mouth. In the older child she places her mouth over the patient's mouth and pinches the nose. She blows until the patient's chest is seen to expand; she then releases her mouth from the patient while expiration takes place. This procedure is repeated 16–18 times/min.

External cardiac massage. The nurse places the heel of one hand over the lower half of the sternum, the other hand is placed on top of it. In infants this technique may be modified by placing one hand behind the infant's chest in order to give a firm base. Keeping the arms straight the nurse will depress the sternum approximately 2.5 cm (1 in.) with a firm rocking movement 70–90 times/min. This action compresses the heart causing blood contained within to be ejected; when pressure is released, the heart refills.

Ideally external cardiac massage and artificial ventilation should be combined. However, if only one nurse is available three or four good ventilations of the lungs should be performed initially, followed by one respiratory ventilation and six cardiac compressions.

Once medical aid arrives, cardiac massage and ventilation will be taken over by the resuscitation team. If possible the head of the bed or cot will be removed to allow free access and a fracture board placed underneath the mattress. An intravenous infusion will also be set up to enable the following drugs to be given.

Sodium bicarbonate 8.4% to counteract metabolic acidosis, calcium gluconate 2%, adrenaline 1:10 000.

Isoprenaline (vasopressor) to sustain the blood pressure.

Effective resuscitation produces a palpable pulse in the carotid and femoral arteries. A pink colour returns to the face and spontaneous respirations and consciousness will return.

Safety measures in hospital

Restrainers and cot sides. In hospital special precautions have to be taken for the child's safety. This is not only for the child's sake, but also because the health authority can be held responsible for any accident, and considerable compensation may have to be paid out of public funds.

Cot sides. These should never be left down not only to stop a child falling out, but also to prevent an active toddler from climbing back in and falling out later. When making the bed of a young child he is best lifted out or else a nurse should be on either side of the cot while the sides are down, or only one side let down at a time. A toddler can roll over with amazing rapidity and fall out on the far side. Bed trays left in position invite the child to climb on to them and make an otherwise adequate cot side low enough for him to fall over.

The vertical bars on cot sides should be no more than 8 cm (3 in.) apart.

Restrainers. The use of restrainers for children at whatever time of the day or night should seldom be necessary and they should only be applied when there is no other method of managing the child while he is undergoing some form of investigation or treatment, or occasionally as a protective measure to prevent the child from injuring himself. The presence of a parent may in some cases eliminate the need for restrainers but it is very important to ensure that the parent does not leave without the staff knowing, because sometimes cot sides are inadvertently left down or the unattended child sometimes may be otherwise at risk. Restrainers should never be used routinely and should only be used as the result of a deliberate decision of the ward sister or deputy and of the consultant or member of the medical staff to whom he has delegated this responsibility. If used, restrainers should be put on with the child's cooperation as part of the process of being dressed. When put on for the first time, the mother may be asked to be present and the cooperation of both mother and child enlisted. The right approach will allay feelings of anger and frustration and will avoid psychological trauma to the young patient.

Restrainers may sometimes have to be applied when there is no other method of managing the child while undergoing some form of investigation or treatment.

Improvised restrainers must never be used (e.g. a harness made from bandages). The best restrainers consist of a close-fitting waistcoat which fastens down the back. The ties, made of webbing, should be secured to the rigid, horizontal part of the cot frame and never to the movable cot sides. The ties should be released when the child is asleep, to exclude danger from strangulation, and be long enough to allow changes of position.

In certain cases it is necessary to prevent children from touching their mouth or face as, for instance, after operation for cleft lip or strabismus. Simple splints can be made from wooden tongue depressors or from a piece of foam latex rolled round the arm, alternatively a roll of corrugated cardboard can be used. These restrainers are known as elbow splints and are applied with light, open-woven bandages. The bandage should first be carried round the child's arm, preferably over a sleeve, and then the well-padded splint is incorporated in the following turns of the bandage. If this is not done, bandage and splint are liable to slip off like a cylinder. For wrists and ankles special restrainers can be made. Alternatively a crêpe bandage tied with a clove hitch may be used. Tubular gauze is another simple alternative. Infants are sometimes wrapped firmly in a blanket to avoid movement during procedures such as subdural tap or taking of venous blood (Fig. 13). Whatever restraint is used, it must be released at least at 4-hourly intervals to allow free movement under supervision.

Prevention of accidents in hospital

Whenever possible children should be allowed to be up and about, rather than kept in bed. This places an extra burden of responsibility on the hospital staff.

The child who presents the greatest problem is the toddler. No equipment left standing about is safe from their urge for adventure. They enjoy opening and closing doors, and easily get their fingers caught. Any unguarded electrical point lends itself to investigation, and milk and other drinks are upset for the mere fun of it.

Children's wards should be as homely as possible and untidiness will never worry an understanding ward sister. But she must be able to anticipate danger and prevent accidents by wise precautions. Some of these are mentioned below but many more could be added and others need only be put into effect when circumstances warrant them.

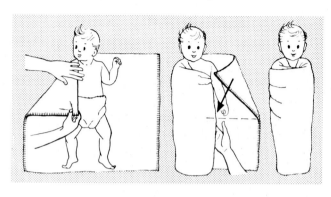

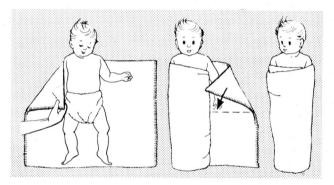

Fig. 13. Restraining the patient.

Very young children should never be allowed out of sight, and objects which may cause accidents should be removed or suitably guarded. These include: sterilizers, radiators, lamps and light switches, thermometers, pots and bottles containing pills, lotions or medicines. All windows should have window-guards and the hot water taps in the bathrooms should be detachable and hung out of the children's reach. Children should never be left unaccompanied in the bathroom and neither bathrooms nor lavatories should have bolts or keys. Drinking glasses and

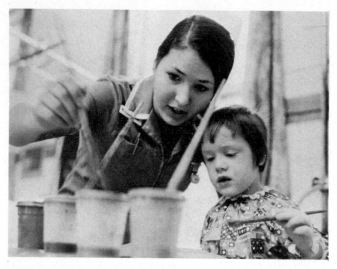

Fig. 14. Painting whilst confined to bed can be fun and absorbing for the young patient.

sharp feeding utensils are unsuitable for the very young and no chipped equipment must ever be allowed in a children's ward. Drinks should be just the right temperature, for a toddler will not wait to test a drink set before him but will eagerly immerse his entire face in a cup. Infants under a year should never be given a soft pillow and are usually best left without any pillows at all. If pillows have to be used they should be small, firm ones or the mattress should be raised by placing a pillow underneath it.

Electrical equipment should never be used unless a nurse can remain with the child for the entire time. Toys should be chosen for their safety, and sharp, protruding corners or wires removed. *Mechanical toys which give off sparks are as dangerous in an oxygen tent as the striking of a match*, and watch must be kept on the type of toy given to children nursed in a tent.

Before taking a rectal temperature the bulb of the thermometer should be inspected and the nurse should keep a firm, restraining hand on the child to avoid sudden movement. Safety pins should be used only where absolutely necessary and should always be left closed when not in use. In many instances a piece of strapping, a tape or a stitch with needle and thread replace safety pins very satisfactorily. Finally, two nurses must always be present when injections are given, as even an apparently reliable 10-year-old may suddenly lose control of himself and move, or grasp a nurse's hand, thus breaking the needle.

Any accident should be reported at once and all details recorded. The parents should be told about it when they next visit, even if the accident was a trivial one.

SICK CHILDREN AT HOME

Wherever it is possible, children should be treated in their own homes under the care of the family doctor, with help from the services of the local authority and attention at the hospital outpatient department if necessary (HM (71) 22).

Nursing the child at home may tax the parents considerably, particularly if they have more than one child to care for. Few children feel ill enough to want to be quiet and inactive for any length of time. Most will want to do things, see what is going on and demand constant company. The mother's work will probably be much reduced if she brings the sick child into the living-room adjoining the kitchen, where she herself has to spend a good deal of time. Often this also means a ground-floor room with a more interesting view out of the window, a saving in heating and far less expenditure on the mother's energy with fewer journeys up and down stairs.

When the sick child is being cared for at home the mother may require advice for certain situations. The following are very basic to the nurse used to working in the well-equipped children's ward, but will prove helpful to the mother seeking guidance.

When to seek medical advice

When to seek medical advice is a constant worry to parents since general practitioners are particularly busy people. It is always best to call him before 10 a.m., and the mother should be able to give a brief description of the illness. Advice should always be sought the same day for the drowsy, irritable child with a headache or earache. Also for the child with any breathing difficulty and for the child of any age with vomiting, pain and diarrhoea, when it is important that the mother should know not to give an aperient. If the child has unexplained bruising or any signs of bleeding the doctor's guidance should be sought. This also applies to the very young child under the age of 6 months whenever he is poorly, refusing feeds or showing any other unusual signs. A child can be very ill without a raised temperature—his health should always be considered in relation to how he looks, any change of behaviour, what he complains of and the appearance of his urine and stools. When a child is ill no observation is too minor to be reported to the doctor, indeed some small symptom noted by the mother will often be most helpful to the doctor in making a diagnosis. Every mother should get to know her family doctor, the health visitor as well as the district nursing sisters who are often attached to group practices in order that she can feel able to seek advice whenever worried.

Medicine cabinets

Medicine cabinets should always be kept locked and well out of the child's reach. All tablets should be kept in child-resistant containers that are now available. All medications in current family use must be clearly labelled. Once a course of treatment is complete any medicines left over should be flushed away down the sink, unless the doctor has particularly suggested that they be retained. There are now some medicine cabinets available with in-built lights—these are more expensive but are the safest, so that when medicines have to be given at night (and often in a hurry) the labels can be clearly read.

First-aid boxes

All homes should maintain a first-aid box that can also be taken with the family when they go on holiday. A basic list should include:

Small pair of scissors with rounded ends.
Tweezers for removing splinters.
Safety pins.
Small stock of sterile packed dressings in assorted sizes.
Roller bandages in 1″ and 2″ (2.5 and 5.0 cm) widths.
A triangular bandage.
Small roll of cotton wool.
Small roll of adhesive tape.
Box of adhesive strip dressings.
Jar of Vaseline.
Antihistamine cream for insect bites.
Antiseptic lotion.
Protective cream for minor burns.

Occupational play activities

There is no need to spend money on toys or books. Indeed there is the obvious danger of spoiling the child who may come to expect gifts every time he is off-colour. Here are a few suggestions, inexpensive, and yet perfectly capable of serving their purpose admirably.

Ages 9–18 months. Magazines and comics to tear up, as well as to look at; simple toys that can be taken apart; balloons, teddy-bears or dolls with various rags to dress and undress; simple rattles made from well-sealed tins filled with pieces of wood (this will make just enough noise without deafening the family); wireless and record players if available with children's records of music and stories.

18 months to 3 years. Old Christmas cards and magazines; large beads to string; crayons; hollow blocks and other building-bricks; a small aquarium or a budgerigar. A bird table just outside the window that can easily be seen by the patient; jigsaw puzzles or picture trays, bought or home made; conkers, daisies and other flowers to play with and examine; percussion instruments.

3–5 years. Beads and conkers (through which father has made a hole); sewing cards with large, blunt needles and coloured thread; rags and bandages to dress and nurse dolls; a nurse's outfit; a doll's tea or cookery set; glove-puppets (home-made).

Dinkie toys; matchboxes with which to build; simple construction toys; interlocking bricks.

Blunt, round-ended scissors; coloured paper; gummed shapes; a scribbling pad; crayons.

5–8 years. Mother's button box to tidy (have a supply of matchboxes); cut-out dolls; dish-cloth yarn and thick needles for knitting dish-cloths for favourite aunts; loosely woven dish-cloths as a foundation for weaving with coloured wools and bodkin. Cotton-reels with four nails at one end for french knitting, coloured wool and a blunt knitting needle.

A book of trains and engines; old motoring and fishing magazines.

Tracing paper and pencils; a magnet; an old watch; a kaleidoscope; milk bottle tops to make mosaic patterns, mould or string up into 'mobiles'.

Matchboxes to build or cover in coloured paper; paints and colouring books; bits of felt or dyed lint and scissors to cut out shapes and for picture making; Plasticine; letter and number cards; toy money. Small squares of lint stuck to figures cut out of magazines, fluffy side outwards, can be made to adhere to a board covered with lint or felt.

Pipe cleaners and large beads can be made into animals and other figures. A thick notebook can be used to make into a diary (words and drawings).

8–12 years. Scissors and thin paper for cutting out strips of people or animals and doilies by folding the paper before cutting and leaving a small piece of the contour uncut to form the link after unfolding; make-up to experiment with; making masks and puppets.

Marbles; packets of inexpensive stamps, a geographical atlas and a notebook for starting a stamp collection. A mirror to play with reflections of light or sunshine; playing cards; an encyclopaedia; 'hobby' books.

Portable T.V.; pop records/cassettes and a player.

A few points to be remembered

1. Protective sheets may be necessary to prevent undue soiling of the top sheet and blankets.

2. Supply a good steady surface such as a tray.

3. Sick children tire quickly, and toys and occupations will need frequent changing.

4. Big or complex toys tire a child more easily than small, simple toys which can easily be changed.

5. A toy enjoyed today may be boring tomorrow.

6. Needless to say the toys given for the various age groups will please older or younger children. It is usually possible to ask friends or neighbours for the loan of books, jigsaws or other toys no longer needed by their own children (some will be only too glad to pass them on for good). The same applies to magazines, scraps of material and gramophone records.

7. The charm of any of these toys and occupations will fade quickly if all are left lying around all the time. Their value is greatly enhanced and their interest doubled if they are tidied away regularly to be brought out again another time.

8. Toys from children who have had an infectious complaint should, of course, be disinfected or destroyed in due course.

Toy libraries

Advise parents to make contact with the nearest Toy Library by writing to:

Toy Libraries Association,
    Seabrook House,
        Wyllyotts Manor, Darkes Lane,
            Potters Bar,
                Herts. EN6 2HL

A Toy Library provides good quality toys which may be borrowed and taken home. See Appendix 2, p. 396.

Preparing for hospital

Sometimes the sick child at home will need to be admitted to hospital and the nurse's advice will often be sought by parents as to how their child should be prepared for this stay. Children should always be told about hospitals, doctors and nurses, from an early age, just as they are prepared for other experiences of life such as going to school. For the emergency admission it is obviously too late for detailed preparation, but the nurse will remember the child's need for comfort and security and that all questions should be answered honestly and directly without giving more detail than the child can understand. For the child on the waiting list to be admitted, the time can be usefully spent in preparing for his admission. Some hospitals produce their own admission booklets which give helpful details about the ward routine and the facilities available. Often a comic or colouring section is included which helps the child to feel that this really is for him. There are also several books that can be bought, or borrowed from the local library.

CARE OF THE DYING CHILD

The care of children suffering from a terminal illness calls for some of the nurse's finest qualities and there is probably no situation which taxes her emotions more severely, nor any other groups of illnesses which she would more sincerely wish to give of her best, both in the care of the patient and by offering mental and spiritual help and comfort to the parents.

Once the terminal condition has been recognized, the parents will want to ask innumerable questions of every person in the hope of getting some understandable information. These will often be repetitive and far seeking, as the parents will be wanting some explanation as to why this should happen to their child. It is best to allow only the smallest possible number of people to discuss the treatment and care, as doubts may arise even if merely different words are used to describe the same thing. Any information given should be consistent and it is often possible to lead up to the subject of a hopeless outcome in several separate conversations. Parents often sense what will have to be said and some will ask a direct question. An honest answer is the only right one in such a case but at the same time the parents can be assured that everything possible will be done to relieve pain and keep suffering to a minimum.

The child, too, will need to know something of his illness, although a great deal will depend upon his age and understanding. In order to help maintain his trust in the medical and nursing staff it is important that information is not withheld from the child. Children rarely ask outright, 'Am I going to die?' but if the nurse finds herself in this situation she should first ascertain what the child means by dying. Children at different stages of development have different ideas, fantasies and experiences. One way of handling this sort of situation is to convey, gradually, the idea of the long-term nature of the illness. That it is not an illness or disorder that can be treated straight away and finished with, but it has an up and down course that cannot be measured in a day or a week. This explanation will relieve the child's anxiety and enable him to anticipate and understand when he has bad days.

Children should also be told whenever there are changes in their medication or treatment. Pain should never be denied and the nurse should never say, 'It won't hurt' when it will, or, 'Don't be a cry baby' when an older child has recourse to tears. But, rather, when a child asks 'Will it hurt?' the nurse should say 'It does hurt a bit, but I'll be very quick, and it will hurt as little as I can make it.' Encourage the child to count as the injection or treatment is carried out, 1 . . . 2 . . . 3, which will help the child to settle and to anticipate the end.

Parents should be with their child as much as they wish, and should be allowed and encouraged to do those things for the child which only a mother or father know how to do. As a rule it is kinder to keep the child in the general ward rather than in a side ward, unless the final weariness becomes too much for him, or his family particularly request it.

Little treats, such as food brought from home, an unusual visit to another part of the hospital or week-end visit at home should be allowed without fear of 'spoiling the child'. The visit of a granny, a beloved teacher or the family vicar should always be permitted.

Children with malignant or terminal illnesses often develop curious fancies, one typical one is the desire to have 'A special meal in the middle of the night'. No nurse should be too busy or too rigid in her routine to grant such a request.

No child should be allowed to die alone. Anticipation of impending death is one of the nurse's primary duties and she should always ensure that members of the family are present if they wish to be. When all is over, those nearest to the child should be left alone for a few moments by the bedside and then led away with quiet, sympathetic firmness. It is commonsense kindness to ensure some rest by giving the parents, with the permission of the attending medical officer, one dose of sleeping tablet to be taken when they reach home.

Last offices

The general procedure of carrying out the last offices differs little from that customary for adults. Detail may, however, be adapted to suit the special cases. Unless the relatives have brought a little gown and socks, a plain white cotton gown or shroud is supplied by the hospital. This should be sufficiently long to cover the feet. If the jaw is inclined to drop, 2.5- to 3-cm bandage, still rolled up as supplied, can be used as a prop between chin and sternum and camouflaged by the gown. This is particularly easily done with infants whose necks are short. With young infants the knees may be drawn up, and they should be straightened by bandaging, some cotton wool being placed between the prominences of the knees to avoid marking the skin. The child's hands are placed together with the fingers interlaced, holding a little white flower. If the arms tend to sag, a roll of cotton wool or a rolled-up napkin can be placed underneath the elbows beside the body to support their weight. The face is covered with a square of gauze or an embroidered handkerchief reserved for the purpose. After securing the body in a sheet, a pall is placed over it and it is carried to the mortuary. Fresh flowers should be placed in the chapel and a light is left burning until the body is removed for burial.

Personal belongings or toys are parcelled up in the usual way but occasionally the parents appreciate the suggestion that a beloved toy should be left with the child.

Answering the questions of other children in the ward about the sudden disappearance of a patient or the inevitable disturbance caused by a death may not be easy. Psychologists are not yet agreed as to what is the best way of dealing with the problem and no two children are likely to react in the same manner, though they will all sense that something unusual has taken place. In the majority of cases it is probably best to state the truth simply, as for instance 'Johnny was so weak he fell asleep and will not wake up again because God has taken him to heaven'. But the nurse should also add immediately—'this will not happen to you—you are not weak, are you?', or words to that effect. As a rule children will be satisfied with this straightforward, honest statement.

Talking about death with children, particularly with those who are terminally ill, is important. Not to do so isolates them from comfort. Not to talk to them about the death of others hinders their development and curiosity.

Raimbault has found that children know about and understand death early in life. They understand the concept much as in the way adults do, i.e. that dead persons disappear from daily life and that their body is elsewhere—a grave, coffin or cemetery. Usually they see death as an endless sort of sleep and as the end of thought. They also look for the reasons why death occurs: illness, handicap, wishes for death or despair.

Many hospitals have the service of a Chaplain available. Whether normally religious or not, most people find it helpful to talk to him at this time and he should always be called. A sympathetic nurse will soon sense what kind of comfort will be of best help to each individual parent. Often the parents have been so preoccupied with their dying child and their impending loss that they have, for the time being, hardly given a thought to their other children at home. This is positive comfort and may be very helpful as it reminds the parents that their responsibilities have not come to an end and that there is much purpose left for them in life. A reminder that death is releasing their child from suffering or from an invalid life is a comfort which may also help. In all instances it is possible to remind parents that children probably lack the apprehension and fear an adult may feel and that their passing is thus made a great deal easier for the parents to come to accept.

The parents' wishes as regards religious observances and orthodox rites should be ascertained and the necessary arrangements made in good time. The nurse should be familiar with the practice of other denominations as well as her own, and all children should be christened, confirmed or given the last rites or any other religious observances as may be wished by the child's family.

HELEN'S BLUE DRESS

Helen's story
by her mother

Helen in hospital

My younger daughter Helen was found to have some hearing loss and an admission was arranged for her adenoids to be removed and grommits to be inserted in her ears. She was not quite three at the time so I asked to stay with her.

Preparation

I visited the ward in advance and talked to the Sister, but did not tell Helen anything until a few days before the admission. We played a few hospital games and I tried to explain that she would have a 'special sleep' when the doctor would put little tubes in her ears to help her to hear better. I did not feel it necessary to mention the adenoids, having checked that she would not feel any pain afterwards. I was glad that I knew in advance that I could stay and that I would be with her for the anaesthetic so that my explanations could be truthful and reassuring. I went into very little detail as I knew Helen was not old enough to take in much and that it would be better for me to explain as we went along.

Admission to the ward

After seeing the doctor we were taken to the ward and shown the cubicle where we were to stay. Helen settled in very happily. I was glad to have the cubicle as it was easier to keep to Helen's home routine and to have peace and quiet when we needed it. I was relieved as well to be able to lie down on my bed when Helen had her rests.

The first day passed uneventfully, apart from the weighing. Helen was asked to stand on a platform which wobbled and frightened her. She cried and refused to get back on. The nurse explained why weighing was essential but I did not want Helen to be really upset by a routine procedure and asked if we could go to the outpatient department, where they had scales she was used to. The Sister was called and she came up with the

Text continued on p. 104

Nursing notes and comments

Helen in hospital

The National Child Development Study showed that no less than 53% of the Nation's children will have been admitted to hospital by the age of 7.

Babies and young children, especially those under the age of 5, need their mother or father to stay with them in hospital if they should be admitted for any reason.

Preparation

Ann Hales-Tooke writes in 'Children in Hospital: The Parents' View' that it is never too early to start talking to small children about hospital, pointing out the big building in the centre of town where the ambulance goes. Learning about hospital and what happens there can be seen as part of the education for life.

A visit to the ward can allay many fears of both parent and child. They should be shown the ward geography, questions should be answered and they should be introduced to staff on the ward, e.g. the playleader, and generally made to feel welcome.

A hospital booklet which provides information for both parent and child can be read aloud and will be helpful. Remember to advise parents of the need to bring along their child's favourite toy or comforter even if it is a scruffy old blanket. The parents themselves should also be advised to bring along some reading material or some knitting because there may be moments when their child is asleep and they need something to occupy themselves. The parents will also need their own toilet articles, nightwear etc.

Admission to the ward

Ideally, resident parents should be offered a cubicle to sleep in with their child. If this is not possible a camp bed should be offered and placed either alongside the child's cot or in the nearby parents' room.

Whenever a parent is resident they should be made to feel 'at home' and introduced to other resident parents in the ward by the nurse. The ward routine with details of doctor's rounds should be explained and the need for any special arrangements such as when the mother may use the bathroom and where to go for meals or to make the occasional cup of tea. The parent should also be told that if she wishes to go out for a short period, perhaps shopping, she should inform the assigned nurse for her child or the nurse in charge of the ward.

Text continued on p. 105

very sensible idea of weighing me holding Helen and then me alone.

I had a five-year-old daughter and a 17-year-old foster son at home. Luckily my husband was able to leave work early to collect Kate from school and come to the hospital to take over from me. I then went home with Kate to put her to bed and spend time with Simon before returning to the hospital to sleep. Kate seemed to enjoy having so much time on her own with me and was in no way upset, but I certainly found it very tiring coping with home chores as well. On the other hand, I did not get bored or 'institutionalized' by staying constantly in the ward.

Pre-operatively

Helen went to bed quite happily in her cot and slept well. I was glad I was beside her to give her a glucose drink in the night. The following morning I bathed her and tried to put on the operating gown which was unfortunately much too large. Helen refused completely to have it on so I put her in her dressing gown for the time being.

She was given a drink of Vallergan but became very 'high' prancing round the cubicle with the vomit bowl as a 'hat'. The Atropine was given by injection in her thigh while I held her on my knee. Unfortunately I did not hold her tightly enough and she got her arm free, knocking the syringe out of the nurse's hand. The injection had to be given again and I felt guilty and incompetent.

Helen quickly fell soundly asleep in my arms. I then tried to slip on the operating gown, but Helen woke, refused angrily to have anything to do with it and insisted on wearing her favourite blue dress. I was anxious to keep her as calm as possible so I put it on, hoping to change it later. As it happened she was operated on still wearing it.

Helen stayed wide awake and insisted I carry her around the ward. A trolley arrived at the appointed time but of course I carried her, talking quite happily until we reached the anaesthetic room. I had asked to hold her until she was unconscious, but was told I must put her on the trolley. She started to cry when I did so but I calmed her and she was quickly unconscious. I left immediately and waited on the ward.

Post-operatively

The Sister fetched me to the recovery room. Helen was coming round, fighting and struggling. For the next 15 min I had to hold her in my arms. If I tried to put her in her cot she would start to fight again. Eventually she fell more deeply asleep and I could put her down.

Helen vomited blood four times during the day. I was a bit worried the first time until I could check with a nurse how much was normal. Helen was not upset, however, and each time fell quickly asleep again. Very soon after

Text continued on p. 106

The parent should be encouraged, as far as the child's condition allows, to take part in the care of the child, helping to maintain fluid balance charts, giving medicines and assisting with washing and feeding as appropriate. In some circumstances the mother may, with instruction, be a very able assistant when holding her child for an injection or a dressing, giving both support and encouragement. Some parents will need to be supported and encouraged to share care in this way.

Pre-operatively

Parents need to be informed and prepared for events in order that they can best help their child. They should also be made aware that there is always a nurse within calling distance if they feel worried. The child's assigned nurse should continue to provide the necessary care according to the care plan which allows adaptation of the ward routine to the child's normal home style as far as is possible.

Post-operatively

Getting away from the ward for a break or a meal can be very difficult if your child does not want you to go. When a child is very ill or recovering from an operation, the parent may feel happier just to stay by the bed and the nurse should recognize this need. In this case, if meals are not provided for parents on the ward, a system should be devised, as in this case, to ensure that the parent is sufficiently sustained and nourished (DS 218/72).

It is difficult to understand why siblings are not allowed to visit the

Text continued on p. 107

coming round, she noticed a plaster on her hand and demanded that I take it off. She recalled this incident later and I realized how aware she had in fact been and was glad I was there as soon as she recovered consciousness.

I did not want to leave Helen to go to the nurse's canteen for a meal as I had no idea when she might vomit. I was glad to be able to make tea in the kitchen close by and very pleased when a nurse offered to get sandwiches for me when she herself went to lunch. The staff were very understanding and allowed me to keep snacks in the ward kitchen for those times when Helen did not want me to leave her. On other occasions I was glad of a chance to leave the ward for a while.

Helen recovered quickly from her operation and we both enjoyed the rest of our stay. I had no chance to get bored as there was no playleader for the ward and I quickly became involved in helping in the playroom. I could see how difficult it was for the nurses to find time to keep equipment in order and I was glad of the things I had brought from home. I liked spending time with the other children, but it was difficult to get away when Helen wanted me to herself. One six-year-old girl in particular attached herself to me. She was desperately miserable when her mother was not there and followed me around from the time I got up.

There was a rule that no brothers or sisters under 12 could visit but towards the end of Helen's stay this was relaxed and I could bring Kate onto the ward for short periods.

Return home

Helen has no bad memories of her stay in hospital and is still as friendly and trusting of doctors and nurses. She coped well with a subsequent admission when she was seriously ill with a chest infection. Once again I was able to stay and undertake most of her care with the help of the staff.

children's ward. Various studies have shown that their exclusion because of the potential increased risk of infection has not been proven. Equally, though, if healthy children are uncontrolled and boisterous in the ward they may disturb the children who are ill. Written information can give parents advice about making their well child's visit short and frequent, and may suggest that when there are children in a family, they should not all visit at once (HC(76)31). Play facilities should, wherever possible, be provided for the visiting children which will help to reassure and comfort the mother, allowing her to concentrate on the sick child and at the same time making the experience of visiting the hospital to see their sick brother or sister a relatively positive one for the visiting child.

Return home

Some children on return home experience disturbed behaviour for a while particularly if mother has not been able to 'live-in'. This usually takes the form of aggressive behaviour as a response to frustration and anger. Toys may be broken up or books torn. The child may also express his anger by attempting to hit his mother or siblings. The child may also regress and become very clinging towards his mother, not wanting to let her out of his sight even if she needs to go to the bathroom. The older child may experience difficulties on return to school.

These behaviour patterns are usually short-lived but parents should be advised that they may happen and are quite a normal reaction to a painful experience. With this understanding the parents will be able to especially comfort and reassure the child and accept the child's behaviour. In this type of loving environment the child will soon become the child they knew before he went into hospital.

Further reading

GENERAL NURSING COUNCIL (1982) *Aspects of Sick Children's Nursing: A Learning Package*, Sections 2 and 3.

HATCH, D. & SUMBER, E. (1981) *Neonatal Anaesthesia*. London: Edward Arnold.

KUBLER-ROSS, E. (1973) *On Death and Dying*. London: Tavistock Publications.

LONG, R. (1981) *Systematic Nursing Care*. London: Faber & Faber.

MCFARLANE OF LLANDAFF, J. K. (1982) *The Practice of Nursing using the Nursing Process*. London: C. V. Mosby.

ROBERTSON, J. (1979) *Young Children in Hospital*. London: Tavistock Publications.

WELLER, B. F. (1980) *Helping Sick Children Play*. London: Baillière Tindall.

Part II
Problem-solving approach to paediatric nursing care

5 Respiration

Ear, nose and throat conditions are very common in childhood, and may account for much minor illness and frequent admissions to hospital or visits to the outpatient clinic. Repeated attacks of catarrh, otitis media, obstructed breathing and sinusitis may contribute to poor general development and diminish mental alertness; loss of schooling may affect the child psychologically as well as educationally.

For children prone to ear, nose and throat infections and congestion, there are some simple measures which are well worth trying in an attempt at improving the tendency to recurrent infections. Among these are simple but thorough education in nose blowing and encouragement at breathing through the nose. Occasionally simple practices such as allowing the child to sleep with the head lower than the rest of the body may encourage drainage and parents should be made to realize that plenty of fresh air, particularly during the day, is as a rule more beneficial than keeping the child indoors for fear of his catching cold.

THE COMMON COLD

Owing to an infant's small air passages, a cold in infancy can be a serious illness. Nurses must always remember this and avoid going near babies when they themselves have a cold; they should realize that a day off duty may prove a greater degree of conscientiousness than being on duty while they are a source of danger. If a nurse herself has to use a handkerchief, this must be done away from the baby's cot and should be followed by hand-washing and a change of mask.

Very young babies breathe wholly through the nose and find mouth-breathing difficult. Nasal obstruction may therefore interfere considerably with feeding as sucking is made almost impossible.

Complications which may arise from a common cold in infancy include otitis media, pneumonia and gastroenteritis.

LARYNGOSCOPY

When a doctor wants to inspect the larynx, trachea or the vocal cords, or if he wishes to remove secretions such as blood, mucus or vomit by suction, laryngoscopy is performed. With very young infants laryngoscopy can often be done without an anaesthetic; with older children, except in dire emergency, a general anaesthetic is given.

Before being placed on the table the child is securely wrapped in a blanket leaving the neck and upper chest exposed. Laryngoscopy may have to be performed in the neonatal period and for some of the conditions described below.

CHOANAL ATRESIA

Choanal atresia is a congenital abnormality in which the openings at the back of the nose are blocked by plates of tissue. Since the newborn infant has not yet adapted himself to breathing through the mouth, the condition has to be corrected as an urgent surgical measure or the baby will die. As the baby struggles to breathe the lips can be seen to move as in a flutter, a typical sign of this condition. An oral airway is introduced and the obstructing plates pierced by means of a probe. If the condition is unilateral treatment can be delayed until the baby is stronger and the structures involved are less minute. In this case babies should always lie on the affected side to ensure an adequate airway.

CONGENITAL LARYNGEAL STRIDOR

Congenital laryngeal stridor is not a dangerous condition and children usually outgrow it by the age of 1 year or 18 months. Parents, however, are concerned about the noise the child makes on inspiration and about the sucking in of the intercostal spaces. The condition is best observed when the child is crying or when asleep. Congenital abnormalities, such as laryngeal web or papilloma must be excluded as both are dangerous forms of respiratory obstruction, but in the majority of cases the parents can be reassured and told that no treatment is needed although it may take several months for the condition to disappear.

CROUP

Laryngitis stridulosa, or croup, is an acute laryngeal spasm causing the patient to struggle for breath in a sudden attack of dyspnoea. The condition affects children of 3–5 years who are of a nervous disposition. The stridor usually occurs in connection with a cold. In a typical case the child awakens in the middle of the night, apparently struggling for air, sweating profusely and in a state of acute anxiety. The attack may last as long as an hour and is followed by normal sleep. Often the child has no recollection of the episode on waking in the morning. While the attacks are very frightening to the parents, they can be reassured about their harmless nature. A warm drink and a sedative may be helpful, and late, heavy meals should be avoided.

LARYNGOTRACHEITIS

Laryngotracheitis, inflammation of the larynx and trachea, is probably caused by a virus; *Haemophilus influenzae*, haemolytic streptococci and staphylococci are often isolated but are thought to be secondary bacterial invaders. Children most commonly affected are aged between 6 months to 2 years.

The chief manifestations of the disease are respiratory obstruction and inspiratory stridor caused by inflammation and congestion of the respiratory tract. The whole of the larynx and trachea is coated with thick, viscous secretions so that the air passages are narrowed. Adequate oxygen exchange becomes impossible and this leads to serious respiratory difficulties and general exhaustion.

Although pyrexia is occasionally absent, the temperature is usually 39.4°–40°C (103°–104°F). The child look anxious, grey and collapsed, the pulse rate is rapid and the volume poor. An almost incessant cough adds to the exhaustion and leads to extreme restlessness. Respirations rise to 60 or more per min as the child struggles for air, and the intercostal spaces and supraclavicular region are drawn in and the stridor increases.

Treatment

Treatment is required urgently. A humidified atmosphere is beneficial as the moisture prevents the secretions from drying.

Occasionally an emergency tracheostomy may have to be performed as a life-saving measure, and fine judgement and careful observation are needed when caring for the patients as sudden deterioration is common. All necessary equipment for tracheostomy should be at hand, including an electric sucker for the extraction of the viscid mucus.

Nursing management

To procure rest should be one of the prime concerns of the nurse. Well-positioned pillows; frequently turned, loose, comfortable clothing (sometimes nothing beyond a napkin if the child is being nursed in a tent); sponging of hands and face; frequent, small sips of water or a glucose drink and even soothing stroking of the head may help to induce rest and so to preserve the strength of these children. The giving of oral fluids may be difficult, but small quantities should be offered if the child is able to take them.

Careful observation of pulse and respirations should be maintained to detect any increasing signs of respiratory obstruction.

Sedatives should be used with caution and are rarely of much value in the acute stages. A course of intramuscular benzylpenicillin and gentamycin is commenced pending the bacterial results of nose and throat swabs taken on admission. In exceptionally severe infections steroids may be given.

TRACHEOSTOMY

Tracheostomy has to be performed whenever the lumen of the larynx has been so narrowed by disease as to make adequate air entry impossible, or to reduce the 'dead space' within the respiratory tract to increase oxygen exchange.

The trachea is opened by a surgical incision and held open either by dilators or by insertion of a tracheostomy tube . This may happen for several reasons, including:

Congenital abnormalities such as papilloma, laryngeal web or cysts.
Trauma, e.g. oedema following intubation or scalding.
Infections such as diphtheria or laryngotracheitis.
Paralysis, e.g. in anterior poliomyelitis.

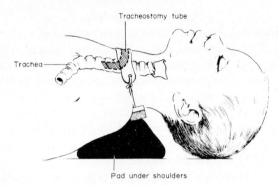

Fig. 15. Tracheostomy. Note position of pad extending the neck.

Signs of obstruction

Distressed respirations, wheezing inspiratory stridor.
Restlessness.
An anxious expression.
Sucking in of the intercostal spaces, the diaphragm, neck muscle, sternal notch and the lower end of the sternum.
An increasing pulse and respiratory rate.
Cyanosis in most, but not all, cases.

With the above signs in mind it should normally be possible to appreciate the impending need for this life-saving procedure and only rarely is an unprepared tracheostomy required. Occasionally a bronchoscopy is done before the tracheostomy and sometimes an endotracheal tube is also passed.

Nursing management

The patient is received back into a warm room. At the conclusion of the operation the tube is fastened securely around the neck by means of tapes. The tapes should always be tied with the neck flexed, as in this position the neck is narrowest. If this is not done the tube may be in danger of slipping out when the head is brought forward. The knot is tied at the side/front of the neck. If white tape is used care must be taken not to confuse with the ties of the child's bib or nightgown: A small pad of polyurethane foam will prevent the tape cutting into the skin.

Nursing action	**Explanation**
To maintain rest. As a rule best maintained by sitting the patient up, well supported with pillows.	Reduced exertion reduces oxygen consumption.
To maintain a clear airway. The chin should be kept off the opening of the tube by extending the neck. This may be achieved by placing a small pillow or pad under the infant's shoulders to allow the head to fall back slightly.	Infants and small children have very short necks.
Fluffy clothing and blankets should be avoided. Clothing worn should be prevented from covering the tube.	To prevent blockage of the tube and inhalation of wisps of fluffy material.
Suction is applied through fine sterile catheters at regular intervals and when required.	To remove secretions.
0.5 ml of 0.9% saline solution may be ordered by the surgeon to be instilled into the tube. After insertion the saline is immediately sucked out. Disposable gloves may be used for this procedure.	To help clear secretions.
Administration of oxygen and humidified air. The patient may be nursed in a humidified environment.	To assist in preventing the secretions drying.
Observe for complications. At first the patient will require an individual nurse.	To ensure a patent airway.
Observation of the colour, the quality of the pulse, and respiratory distress with restlessness.	To ensure blood oxygen level is adequately maintained.

Nursing action	**Explanation**
Listen for audible vocal noise. The obstruction in the tube should, if possible, be removed by suction. If this fails the tube should be removed and the tracheal dilators inserted.	The tube is obstructed and help should be sent for immediately.
Maintaining hydration and nutrition. Frequently small amounts of fluids should be given orally. A light diet as soon as condition permits. Care should be taken to avoid any fluid entering the tube. If swallowing is difficult a nasogastric may be used.	A tracheostomy does not interfere with feeding.
Restraint. Wrist restrainers or elbow splints may be necessary.	To prevent the child handling the tube.
Communication. Speech is impossible and care should be taken to maintain communication by talking to the patient and providing a means whereby a child can indicate his needs, e.g. paper and pencil, or bell.	The tracheostomy tube bypasses the vocal cords and prevents the use of the voice.

Tracheostomy performed in cases of acute illness, as in laryngotracheitis, can often be allowed to close after only a few days by plugging the tube for experimental periods. In cases of congenital abnormalities or neoplasm it may have to be permanent. Parents and children then have to learn how to manage the tube. The patient may be able to lead a fairly normal life.

Removal of tube. After having had a tracheostomy for several days, children are rather apprehensive when the tube is to be removed. It is often helpful to give a sedative before attempting to do so. Occasionally the tube can be best removed while the child is drinking some favourite drink, as at this time normal rhythm between swallowing and breathing is easily established before the young patient is aware of what has been done.

TONSILLITIS

Tonsillitis is most frequently caused by the haemolytic streptococcus, and is common in children. The patient is often severely ill, particularly children under school age.

As children are not always capable of describing pain accurately, they may complain of abdominal pain. Vomiting may be present and it is not easy to exclude acute appendicitis. As the neck is frequently held stiffly, the condition may also be mistaken for meningitis. Often mesenteric adenitis develops simultaneously causing general rigidity and confusing diagnosis still further.

The child is generally ill and fractious. The face is flushed, the temperature perhaps as high as 39.4°C (103°F) and headache may cause him to turn away from the light. Saliva may dribble from the mouth or alternatively the lips are parched and cracked.

When any other conditions have been excluded, a throat swab is taken to determine the causative organism and its sensitivity to drugs. Penicillin, given by injection, is the drug most commonly used.

Nursing management

If admitted to hospital, patients suffering from tonsillitis should be barrier nursed for at least 24 hours after commencing treatment. If there is a high temperature the bedclothes should be light and supported by a bed cradle. An electric fan, well out of reach of the patient, may be used, and tepid sponging may be carried out with the doctor's permission. Mouth toilet, including mouth washes with a mild antiseptic such as glycothymoline or with saline, will help to keep the mouth clean.

Aspirin gargles may relieve the pain and are often given about 20 min before meals to make swallowing easier. As the child is likely to refuse solid food in the early stages of the illness, he should be encouraged to take frequent drinks of cool, bland fluids. Ice-cream is soothing and is often taken eagerly when other foods are refused.

Antibiotics usually make tonsillitis a short illness and the child is greatly improved after 24 hours.

Special points

If nursed in an open ward, these children should never be placed next to others suffering from acute rheumatism, nephritis or congenital heart disease, as streptococcal infections are serious in patients suffering from these conditions.

TONSILLECTOMY AND ADENOIDECTOMY

Operation for the removal of tonsils and adenoids is among the more common surgical procedures in a children's unit. The removal of diseased tonsils and hypertrophied adenoids improves a child's general health, and other illnesses such as recurrent tonsillitis, otitis media, sinusitis and general development can be improved.

Frequently, tonsillectomy or adenoidectomy is performed on children under the age of 5 years. The presence of the mother during the stay in hospital is particularly beneficial to both child and mother and may be the best means to ensure that there are no psychological after effects.

Pre-operative nursing management

Nursing action	Explanation
Temperature, pulse and respiration rate are taken.	To identify any infection that would cause the operation to be postponed.
Long hair is tied back.	To prevent contamination of the operation site.
General preparation for anaesthesia.	

Post-operative nursing management

Position. Nursed on the side with the upper leg bent and upper arm flexed (tonsillectomy position). A pillow in the back assists in maintaining the position until the patient regains full consciousness.

This position prevents any blood trickling down the throat and will ensure it comes out of the mouth.

Observations. Restlessness and noisy respirations together with regular swallowing movements are indications of bleeding. If these symptoms go unnoticed the pulse rate rises and the pulse becomes weaker.

Fresh blood in vomit may be an indication of bleeding.

The temperature is taken 4-hourly in the axilla.

The complication of bleeding post-operatively is due to the highly vascular operation site. Serious haemorrhage necessitates a return to theatre.

The early signs of infection require identification. Mouth breathing post-operatively makes oral temperature recording unreliable.

Relief of pain. Analgesia should be given regularly during the first 12 hours. Aspirin gargles before meals, will ease throat pain during the first few days.

Reduces the incidence of shock, restlessness and haemorrhage. Prevents stiffness of the throat, allowing movement and thus preventing infection.

Maintaining hydration and nutrition. Cool drinks of fruit juice and water should be encouraged in the first 12 hours. A normal diet may be given avoiding hard foods during the first few days.

Drinking prevents the throat from becoming stiff and painful.

Mobility. The child may be sat up after 12 hours, providing observations remain stable, and the hands and face are sponged.

After 24 hours the child should be gradually mobilized.

Discharge. The child may be discharged home after 3–7 days, providing the temperature is normal. The convalescence continues at home avoiding infection and crowded places.

DEAFNESS

Deafness in childhood may be temporary or permanent. Permanent deafness may be congenital nerve deafness caused, e.g. by an attack of rubella in the mother, during the first 12 weeks of pregnancy. Cerebral palsy sufferers often also have an associated nerve deafness.

Among the acquired causes are repeated attacks of otitis media and perforation of the ear drum with subsequent scarring and adhesions. Transitory deafness may be caused by an accumulation of wax, a foreign body in the meatus, meatal boils and blocking of the Eustachian tube due to a cold, sinusitis or adenoids.

Total deafness is rare. Once any doubt about a child's hearing has arisen, no time must be lost in seeking expert advice—a 'wait and see' attitude may prejudice the entire future of the child. Tests to assess the degree of deafness can now be carried out on very young babies at special audiology centres staffed by specialists in the diagnosis of deafness in children. Once the deafness has been confirmed a training and stimulation programme can be planned with the child's parents who will have a great part to play in developing any potential of hearing, speech and intelligence. They should therefore be encouraged to participate in the training from the start. Deaf children should be allowed to mix with those with normal hearing, and education will take place within ordinary schools, with special classes for the benefit of the deaf child.

OTITIS MEDIA

Otitis media is inflammation of the middle ear. In young children the structures of the ear, nose and throat are particularly closely related to one another, and their smallness easily accounts for frequent congestion and blocking and for the spread of infection from one to the other. Otitis media is common as a secondary infection following a common cold, tonsillitis, infections of the mouth, infectious fevers and carious teeth. In babies, the short, straight and rather wide Eustachian tube may even become blocked by vomitus, and special care should be taken with babies suffering from any kind of vomiting.

Signs and symptoms

The onset of otitis media may be insidious and the first signs may be that the young child rolls his head on the pillow, pulls his ear and is abnormally irritable. Pain soon becomes severe, the temperature rises as high as 39.4°C (103°F) and the patient resents being touched. He looks toxic, and diarrhoea, vomiting and convulsions are common. On examination the blood vessels of the ear drum are found to be dilated and congested, the cone of light normally reflected from it is absent, and the usual mobility of the drum is lost. The ear drum may be bulging and opaque owing to the pus which fills the cavity of the middle ear.

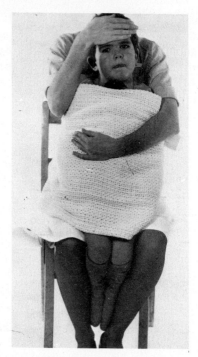

Fig. 16. This comfortable and secure method of holding a child for examination of the mouth and throat is also used for gastric lavage. If the head is turned to one side, this position can also be used for examination of the ear.

Treatment

Penicillin is usually given in large doses. The application of gentle heat may be soothing. Disprin is a useful agent to relieve pain, particularly at night. 1% Ephedrine nasal drops, which have the effect of shrinking the mucosa of the nose and Eustachian tube, may be ordered to promote drainage of secretions.

Grommet tubes

Tiny drainage tubes called Grommet tubes are placed in the ear for drainage. The tubes have small flanges at each end and they act as aerators as well as drains. They are left in situ until the Eustachian tubes, blocked by catarrh, have cleared.

OTORRHOEA

Serous or purulent discharge from the ear may be either acute or chronic. In either case, treatment will consist of three main factors:

Treatment by antibiotics.
Regular, thorough aural toilet by syringing or mopping.
Building up the patient's general health.

Ear mopping

Ear mopping should be painless and is essentially the same in children as in adults. The auditory meatus in young children up to the age of approximately 18 months is of different anatomical shape and in order to straighten it sufficiently to reach the bottom of the meatus when mopping, the pinna should be gently pulled in a backward direction; in older patients hold in a backward and upward direction.

The delicate skin of children easily becomes excoriated by aural discharge. The area around the ear should be gently washed with cotton wool and saline, and zinc ointment or lanolin applied.

MYRINGOPLASTY

Occasionally a long-standing perforation of the ear drum is closed by skin graft. The necessary skin is taken from the upper arm, inner aspect of the thigh, a vein or from the ear. Working with the help of a microscope throughout the operation, the surgeon cleans the ear carefully and removes the upper skin of the tympanic membrane before applying the graft. The graft is kept in position by tiny plastic or nylon sponges, packed tightly into the auditory meatus and left undisturbed for at least 10 days. The operation is very delicate and only about half the cases are entirely successful. If the graft has taken discharges cease and the danger that infection might enter the middle ear is eliminated. Hearing is restored to a useful level.

CLEFT LIP AND CLEFT PALATE

Approximately one baby in every thousand is born with a cleft lip or cleft palate so that most nurses are likely to meet this abnormality in the course of their paediatric experience. Cleft lip and cleft palate are often hereditary and are caused by a failure of development in the first 3 months of pregnancy. Many degrees of severity of this deformity occur and either condition can be present without the other. The cleft may be unilateral or bilateral, it may merely be a small notch in the upper lip, and it can be incomplete or extend deep into the nostrils. If the cleft is centrally placed the deformity is known as hare lip. Cleft palate may involve only the uvula or be a small hole in the soft or hard palate, but more often the cleft extends through both hard palate and soft palate. The cleft may be narrow or wide and may include the alveolar margin and if associated with a bad cleft lip causes an ugly protrusion of the premaxilla bone. In the majority of cases cleft lip is associated with an asymmetry and flattening of the nose.

Cleft lip
General points
   A mother who has a baby with a cleft lip is likely to be

deeply distressed at the time of the birth. This can be greatly relieved if the midwife can show the mother some photographs of similar babies before and after surgical repair. The closure of the cleft lip may help to push back the protruding premaxilla and later produce a better dental arch and a more regular development of the teeth. A small prosthesis achieves the same thing. The operation is usually carried out when the baby is well established and thriving, which is often within a few days of birth.

Cleft lip without cleft of the palate does not often interfere with sucking and in many cases breast-feeding can be carried out successfully. Alternatively, special nipple shields and teats are available and only severe cases of cleft lip and cleft palate need to be spoon-fed from birth. Even then the breasts should be expressed and the milk given to the infant as long as lactation can be maintained. When the cleft is complete, feeding may be very difficult as regurgitation through the nose causes the baby to cough and sneeze. When spoon feeding, the milk should be allowed to run on to the back of the tongue or into the cheek, as this reduces regurgitation through the nose and checks irritation. Upper respiratory tract infections, inhalation pneumonia and otitis media are common.

Babies with cleft palates tend to swallow air during feeding and special care must be taken when 'bringing up the wind'. A little boiled water is often given after feeds to clean the mouth and prevent crusts of milk from forming around the edges of the cleft.

Pre-operative nursing management

Nursing action	Explanation
Pre-operative examination. A photograph taken for record purposes.	For comparison post-operatively.
Nose and throat swabs for culture.	The baby should be free from infection.

Nursing action

Feeding. Feeds should be given by spoon, being careful not to injure the mucous membrane inside the mouth. A special spoon with the sides bent to form a trough is useful.

Boiled water should be given after all feeds.

After feeds the chin should be well dried.

Estimation of haemoglobin.

Parental involvement. Ideally the mother should be resident with her child and participate in the care.

Preparation for theatre. In the usual way.

Explanation

To prevent injury to the suture line feeds are administered post-operatively by spoon.

To reduce the risk of infection of the surgical wound.

To prevent excoriation.

For estimation of blood loss during operation.

The patient benefits from being handled and fed by its own mother.

Post-operative nursing management

Position. The infant is nursed on his side with the foot of the bed raised.

To assist the free drainage of secretions.

Maintaining an airway. Oedema may obstruct the airway, particularly the nasal passages.

Restrainers. Elbow splints are applied, particularly during the semi-conscious phase, or alternatively the child is held by the mother.

To prevent handling of the suture line.

Wound care. Tension on the sutures should be prevented. Sometimes a Logan's bow is applied to prevent tension. Crying should be prevented by frequent picking up and handling.

Tension will cause a widening of the wound line when sutures are removed.

Nursing action	**Explanation**
Toilet of the suture line is carried out regularly and after feeds. The wound is kept dry. Alternate sutures are removed on the 4th and 6th days if catgut sutures are not used.	To prevent infection.
	To reduce scarring.
Feeding. The first feed is given when the infant appears hungry. A normal feeding pattern is then resumed giving the feeds by spoon.	Post-operative feeding problems are unusual.
The baby can be put to breast after the sutures have been removed.	

The child is ready for discharge once the sutures have been removed.

Cleft palate

Repair of cleft palate

The usual age for repair of cleft palate is 12–24 months, i.e. before the child begins to talk, so that any bad habits of speech may be prevented from developing. Children with cleft palates are often late in commencing to talk. Long before this, however, orthodontic treatment may have been started with the intention of moulding the maxilla into a well-shaped arch and to stimulate growth of the under-developed maxilla.

The preparation of the child with a cleft palate for operation differs little from that of preparing for repair of a cleft lip. The post-operative management is also principally the same as described under cleft lip. The oozing of blood from the sutured palate may occur, and the vomiting of stale blood.

Specific care

Ribbon gauze packs may be in situ either side of the palate

and the child should be encouraged not to dislodge them with the tongue. There is a greater danger of the airway becoming obstructed. The elbow splints will be worn for longer periods of time.

For the first 10 days all foods should be liquid or semi-solid and meals should be followed by a drink of plain water to wash down any remains of food. The diet should be rich in vitamins, protein and iron. It is important that neither boiled, hard sweets, nor toffees should be given and this should be explained to the parents.

Speech therapy

Speech therapy is of great importance in promoting early, normal speech. As soon as the post-operative oedema has subsided the nurse can start to play games, such as blowing bubbles and practising the consonants K and T in order to encourage normal articulation. On discharge the child is referred to a speech therapist for assessment, and in some cases the mother can be taught exercises which can be practised at home until such time as the child is old enough to benefit from organized speech therapy.

PIERRE ROBIN SYNDROME

Sometimes babies are seen who have a series of abnormalities, referred to as Pierre Robin syndrome.

These babies have a small, receding mandible (retrognathia), a widely cleft palate and an abnormally small mouth (microstoma). The tongue seems to have insufficient anchorage so that it slips down the back of the throat (glossoptosis). It follows that the tongue obstructs the airway when the baby lies on his back; normal feeding is impossible.

The nursing care of these babies is all-important. The nurse must build up pillows or wedges of polyurethane which make it possible to nurse the baby face down so that the tongue falls forward by gravity. Sometimes a wooden frame or plaster cast can be constructed; tube feeding is usually necessary until the baby weighs about 2 kg (4 lb), but a plate made of acrylic resin may help to occlude the cleft palate during feeding. Sucking should be encouraged, as this strengthens the tongue and develops the mandible.

The surgeon may stitch the tongue to the mandible and cause adhesions to form—Douglas operation—or he may transfix the tongue with wire to prevent it from slipping back. As the baby grows bigger the difficulties resolve themselves sufficiently so as no longer to endanger the child's breathing and life.

Complications include aspiration pneumonia and cyanotic attacks which, if severe, lead to brain damage.

RESPIRATORY TRACT

Young children are very prone to diseases of the respiratory tract, mainly due to the small lumen of the air passages and to their poorly developed immunity to infection.

During infancy and early childhood, respirations are often shallow, rapid, and irregular in rhythm. At birth the baby breathes about 30–40 times/min, by the end of the first year the respiratory rate at rest decreases to approximately 24–30 respirations/min, by the age of two it is 20–24 and by the age of 5 years the respiratory rate is the same as that of an adult.

Respiration

Changes in the rate and depth of respiration occur easily in children and the cause is not always in the respiratory system. Abdominal pain may cause shallow breathing while any increase in the metabolic rate, such as fever, will send the respiration rate up. It is possible to learn much from careful observation of a child's breathing. In obstruction of the air passages, the neck and chest wall can be observed sucking in at the intercostal spaces or the suprasternal notch.

The respiratory rate is best taken when the child is asleep to gain the most accurate results.

Examination of the child

It is usual for a nurse to assist the paediatrician in his examination. It is her duty to see that the patient is comfortable and well supported, with a small blanket at hand to avoid unnecessary exposure. The child who is old enough to understand, should be told what is going to happen and it is usually beneficial to spend a few minutes gaining the child's confidence. He could handle the stethoscope or listen to his own or teddy's chest. The stethoscope should be warmed before use as the touch of a cold object may frighten or arouse protest.

The paediatrician will first watch the child's breathing for depth, regularity, complete and symmetrical expansion of the chest wall, any undue wasting and any drawing in of the intercostal spaces. He will note whether the respirations are abdominal or thoracic and determine the position of the apex beat. By now the child will have gained confidence and only then will the doctor use his stethoscope.

X-ray examination

It is often difficult to obtain good radiographs of young children, but it will help a great deal if someone with whom the patient is familiar can accompany him to the department, if possible arrange for the mother to be present and assist. It is well to remember the fear a child may feel when confronted with a dark, unknown room or with the enormous structure of the X-ray machinery. The X-ray plates and table should be covered with a soft warm material to prevent protesting screams which may make the procedure difficult and unsuccessful.

Positioning of babies and toddlers, particularly when they are feeble and limp or crying, may cause problems. The child cannot be expected to hold his breath during exposure. Often, therefore, more than one picture has to be taken and both lateral and posterio-anterior pictures are required.

Special investigations

Laryngoscopy

When a doctor wants to inspect the larynx, trachea or the vocal cords, or if he wishes to remove secretions such as blood, mucus or vomit by suction, laryngoscopy is performed. With very young infants laryngoscopy can often be done without an anaesthetic; with older children, except in dire emergency, a general anaesthetic is given.

Bronchoscopy

Bronchoscopy may be done for various reasons. At times it may be performed in order to observe the interior and lining of the lung. Pus and viscous secretions may be sucked out and the cause of collapse of the lung may be observed or removed as for instance a foreign body or a tuberculous gland. Tissue may be removed for biopsy examination.

The procedure is the same as for adults, but children are usually given an anaesthetic and preparation is carried out accordingly. The throat may be made insensitive by means of a cocaine or Decicain spray.

Bronchoscopy is not entirely without danger. The small air passages may go into spasm during the procedure causing asphyxia. A drink given before a good swallowing reflex has returned and the effect of the local anaesthetic has worn off, will have serious consequences as fluid may enter the lungs. Approximately 4 hours should elapse between spraying the throat and giving the first drink, 5 ml of water, followed by larger amounts if tolerated.

Bronchography

Preparation of the patient for bronchography should include postural drainage being carried out at night and by a physiotherapist or nurse immediately before the child goes to the X-ray department. This will remove some of the stagnant mucus or pus.

Bronchograms are done in the X-ray department or operating theatre under a general anaesthetic. Premedication should ensure that the child is fast asleep before being moved to unfamiliar surroundings. Radio-opaque substance, usually iodized oil, is introduced into the main bronchus by the passage of a fine catheter over the back of the tongue into the trachea. The child is rotated to allow the dye to flow into the lobes and the radiograph will show the outline of the bronchial tree of selected lobes. Irregular filling will demonstrate abnormalities suspected on clinical grounds and from straight X-ray.

On return to the ward, postural drainage is started almost at once. Thus the danger of the iodized oil, pus or secretions spilling into the healthy parts of the lung is reduced. Frequently, the patient complains of a sore throat after a bronchogram and there may be a productive cough for some days.

The radio-opaque substance used for bronchography contains iodine which may set up sensitivity reactions. Sensitivity tests should be carried out before the procedure and the consent form is signed by the child's parents.

ACUTE BRONCHITIS

Upper respiratory tract infections are very common in

childhood, and may occur in the prodromal period of measles or pertussis. They may be mild or severe. When the inflammation spreads down into the bronchial tree, the patient suffers from bronchitis.

Acute bronchitis most frequently attacks children from overcrowded homes who are ill-nourished and debilitated. It is a common complication of measles or influenza, and children suffering from fibrocystic disease of the pancreas, Down's syndrome or congenital heart defects are particularly prone to this and other chest infections. Allergic bronchitis, a familial condition, may also occur. In younger children the illness remains a serious one.

Signs and symptoms

The child suffering from acute bronchitis looks and feels ill. His cheeks are flushed and his skin and mouth are dry due to a fever of 39.4°–40.6°C (103°–105°F) or more. Respiratory difficulties make him restless and irritable. The accessory muscles of respiration come into play and the alae nasi may be working. The respiratory rate is increased and the respirations may be shallow due to pleural pain. A cough, harsh and dry at first but later productive, is present throughout the 24 hours and is both an early and an exhausting feature of the illness.

In young children the sputum is swallowed and this may at times lead to gastric irritation and vomiting. Occasionally the mucous secretions form a plug in one of the bronchial tubes causing collapse of a lobe or segment of the lung.

Specific treatment

Oxygen therapy may be of use, provided the atmosphere is kept moist during the early, dry stage of the illness. Steam from a kettle may be used at home to warm and moisten the atmosphere of a room. Humidified oxygen into a tent being the method of choice in hospital.

Drugs

Appropriate antibiotics are given to combat the infection. Drugs to relieve bronchial spasm are used selectively. Cough mixtures and expectorants are rarely of value for children. Nasal drops may be ordered to clear the upper respiratory passages.

Complications

Collapse of one or more sections of the lung, anaemia, and general debility may follow the acute stages of the illness while in young babies diarrhoea and vomiting are frequently associated with it.

Nursing management

As children suffering from acute bronchitis may be incubating measles, they should be isolated from the general ward in a warm, well ventilated cubicle for the first few days. Breathing may be difficult so several pillows should be arranged to give maximum support in a sitting position that the child finds comfortable. Alternatively, the child may be nursed flat, the pillows removed and the foot of the bed raised to promote drainage by gravity. Unless the patient does so himself, the position should be changed frequently so as to move secretions and avoid the formation of mucous plugs. When the secretions are profuse and the patient too weak to cough nasopharyngeal suction will be required.

Humidified air

The objective should be to maintain a circulation of moistened air within an enclosed area, whilst being able to observe the child without obstruction.

The most common method of administration is to release air under pressure through a container of water with a narrow outlet. This creates a vapour which is directed into a tent, incubator or cubicle. The moistened air causes the child's clothing and bedclothes to become damp, requiring them to be changed at intervals for dry ones. Frequent observation of the patient's body temperature and the incubator/tent temperature is required to observe for an increase in temperature that may result from a patient being in an enclosed space. The temperature may fall causing the patient to become cold in the moist atmosphere.

The nurse should be available within the vicinity whilst steam therapy is in progress, unless the mother is staying. As the acute stage of the illness passes the child will require suitable play activities to maintain rest.

Oxygen therapy

Oxygen is given when prescribed by the doctor, unless being used in an emergency situation for resuscitation. It may be dangerous to give oxygen in excessive amounts or in too high a concentration (see p. 53). The amount to be given per minute should be ascertained from the doctor. An accurate flowmeter is required. The usual precautions when giving oxygen apply. The danger from striking a match and smoking does not apply with small children but remains a hazard with parents, visitors and older children. Explosions can result from sparks given off from mechanical toys or nylon clothing and visitors need to be warned of this.

Children soon show signs that they lack oxygen by being restless and looking anxious. The respirations become rapid and gasping and the lips and extremities cyanosed.

Methods of giving oxygen. Not all methods used for giving oxygen to adults are suitable for children. In newborn infants, oxygen given through an endotracheal tube or into an incubator are the most commonly used methods. There are various models of oxygen tents for use at different ages.

Patients with a tracheostomy may have to be given

oxygen. The humidified oxygen can be delivered directly into the tracheostomy tube by means of a polythene catheter or a specially designed collar and fitting. Alternatively, the patient may be nursed in an oxygen tent. Chest physiotherapy is given to assist coughing and the removal of secretions. Clothing should be light and warm.

Coughing may be troublesome, often warm milk and honey are enjoyed and very effective for relief. Fluids should be given freely, but sore throat, trachitis and cough may cause the patient to be reluctant and difficult. For bottle-fed babies the feeds are best given diluted during the acute phase and spoon feeding may prove less exhausting than sucking. The feeds should be small and frequent so as to avoid distension of the stomach and resulting pressure on the diaphragm.

The patient is observed for physiological signs of a deteriorating condition. Temperature, pulse and respirations are taken 4-hourly and any changes reported. The pulse volume and respiratory rate should be observed with special care to detect signs of oxygen shortage. The blood gases will be estimated at regular intervals. Intake and output charts should be kept as the intake may be small and renal output poor. As a rule the illness is acute but of short duration and mouth toilet, treatment of pressure areas and the care of bowels present few problems.

BRONCHIECTASIS

Bronchiectasis is a dilatation of the bronchi and bronchioles, resulting from the blockage of a bronchus, and may occur as a result of repeated chest infections, pertussis or measles. One or several sections of the lung may be involved. Additionally, a swallowed foreign body that has 'gone the wrong way', e.g. a peanut, resulting in bronchial obstruction will lead to bronchiectasis. It is inadvisable to give peanuts to young children in view of this danger.

Children so affected are pale, undernourished, under-developed and generally suffer from poor health. They usually have chronic upper respiratory tract infections and frequently the mother gives a history of several attacks of otitis media, sinusitis and chronic cough. In its severest form, which fortunately is now being seen far less than some years ago, clubbing of fingers may be present. The teeth may be carious and the tongue coated. Halitosis is common and these children usually breathe through their mouths on account of the chronic nasal obstruction which is present. Hearing is frequently impaired. The chest wall may be deformed, there is shortness of breath and often a low-grade fever. Sputum is profuse, greenish, purulent and very offensive in advanced cases. The younger children are inclined to swallow the sputum, which causes gastric irritation and loss of appetite. Interrupted schooling, the result of frequent admissions to hospital, adds to the impression of dullness so often seen in these children.

Straight radiographs and bronchograms are done to confirm the clinical diagnosis. The sputum is sent for culture and for tests to determine the sensitivity to various drugs of any organisms present. White blood counts, blood sedimentation rate, Mantoux test and sinus X-ray are performed and estimations of peak air flow and inspiratory–expiratory volumes are made. Antrum washout may be necessary for the frequently associated sinus infection, and dental treatment should be given when indicated.

The patient is treated with postural drainage of the lungs and intensive chest physiotherapy. Nose drops are some-times useful for clearing phlegm before postural drainage is attempted.

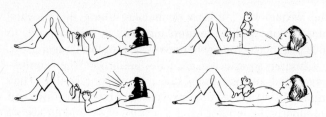

Fig. 17. Breathing exercises can be made to be fun.

Postural drainage of the lungs. When the internal passages become inflamed, the membranes lining the lungs produce mucus or phlegm. If the phlegm becomes too thick or too much, it may hinder recovery by blocking the passages. Usually phlegm is coughed up and spat out, though children often swallow it without very much harm. If the phlegm is very thick, it cannot be brought up so easily and may stagnate. Postural drainage is to remedy this. From the physiotherapist, nurses and parents can learn to understand the positions which allow for maximum drainage of the affected lobe.

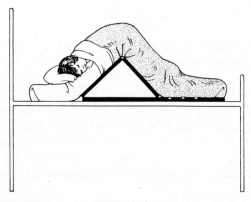

Fig. 18. If a child tips over with hips above the head, it helps the phlegm to run out of the chest.

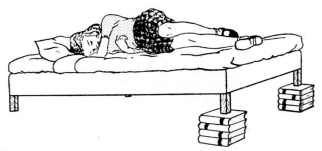

Fig. 19. Postural drainage. To clear the middle lobe you lie on your left side; to clear the left you lie on your right side.

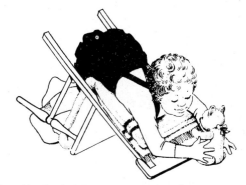

Fig. 20. A position for draining the right and lower left lobes.

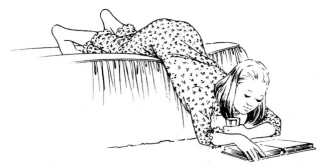

Fig. 21. Postural drainage. Keep this position for 10 minutes three times a day following a hot drink.

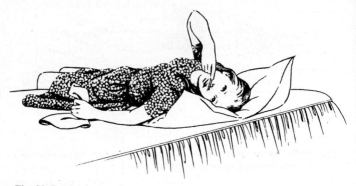

Fig. 22. Putting in nose drops.

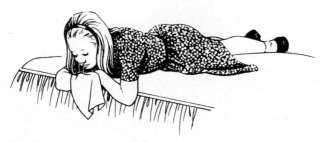

Fig. 23. After waiting half a minute, allow the nose drops and phlegm to run out.

LOBAR PNEUMONIA

Various organisms may be responsible for causing the lungs to become infected and setting up inflammation. In lobar pneumonia one or several lobes of the lung may be affected. Lobar pneumonia rarely affects young infants. The patients are, as a rule, otherwise healthy, active children who are taken ill with great suddenness. They appear very ill with little warning though occasionally an attack of vomiting or a convulsion may herald the illness.

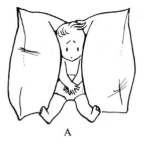 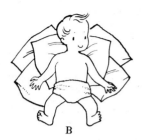

A   B

Fig. 24. Correct use of pillows in upper respiratory tract infections. (A)
Wrong: **Young children should never be given large, soft pillows as there
is a danger of suffocation and overheating. (B)** *Right*: **The pillows are
arranged to allow air to circulate, important in cases with pyrexia, and to
allow for full expansion of the chest on inspiration.**

Nursing management

Nursing action	Explanation
The child's temperature will be measured 4-hourly, the bedclothes cradled and the room temperature controlled. An electric fan can assist in bringing down the body temperature.	The temperature rises rapidly to 39.4°C.
Sponging of face and hands will be soothing.	Will promote patient comfort.
Nursed sitting up, supported by firm pillows, or alternatively a baby chair may be used for small children.	Breathing is shallow and rapid.
Deep breathing exercises with encouragement to bring up sputum when cough becomes productive.	Painful cough may cause cough to be suppressed and prevent good expansion of lungs. May have referred abdominal pain.
Administration of oxygen may be required.	If cyanosis present and respirations laboured.

Nursing action	Explanation
Copious oral fluids monitored on a fluid balance chart.	The high fever will cause urinary output to be low and urine concentrated.
Mouth, lips and pressure areas treated at regular intervals.	The fever causes the mouth and skin to be hot and dry.
Administration of antibiotics as prescribed according to sensitivity of the organisms.	Bacterial infections respond well to broad spectrum antibiotics.

BRONCHOPNEUMONIA

In contrast to lobar pneumonia, bronchopneumonia most commonly affects babies and children who are already weak and debilitated and this is one of the reasons why it is by far the more severe of the two illnesses. It often affects very young infants and is a fairly common complication of whooping cough, measles, severe burns and fibrocystic disease of the pancreas.

Occasionally the onset is acute but more often there is a history of an apparently harmless cold for 2 or 3 days. Then cough and fever develop and the child soon appears to be severely ill. Convulsions are common at the onset.

Nursing management

Most of the nursing points applicable to lobar pneumonia are the same for bronchopneumonia. It is important that all treatment and nursing management are planned to make any disturbance of the patient as infrequent and brief as possible.

In addition to the use of antibiotics the treatment may include digitalis preparations if there is evidence of cardiac failure.

Complications

In spite of modern therapy bronchopneumonia continues to be a serious illness. As large areas of the lung are congested, pulmonary circulation is restricted causing considerable strain on the infant's heart. One or more lung segments may collapse, later leading to bronchiectasis. Other complications include convulsions, diarrhoea and vomiting, and pleurisy.

Convalescence

Following discharge the child may not be quite ready to return to school. If possible the parents should be encouraged to take a family holiday to build up general health and resistance. Medical supervision should continue until the doctor is satisfied that the lungs are once more fully expanded.

The family health visitor and/or school nurse should be informed prior to discharge.

PLEURISY

When the pleura become inflamed, as may happen as a complication of pneumonia, the condition is known as pleurisy.

As the inflammation spreads from the lungs, the two layers of pleura rub against each other and cause severe pain. The child restricts both breathing and coughing to a minimum on account of the pain, and this causes both rapid and shallow respirations. He may also lean towards the affected side in an attempt to splint and immobilize it. Sometimes the pain is referred to the iliac fossa and may cause the doctor to suspect acute appendicitis. As an effusion forms, the inflamed surfaces are separated and the pain subsides.

A Mantoux test and a radiograph of the chest must be taken to exclude tuberculosis and, if an effusion is present, some fluid should be sent for examination and culture.

Treatment

Treatment of the underlying cause is often all that is required. In mild cases the effusion is absorbed spontaneously but when it causes respiratory distress or displaces the heart and mediastinum, chest aspiration must be performed. In either case fibrous adhesions form and often show up on routine radiographs throughout the patient's life. Apart from this, recovery can be complete but a good follow-up and prolonged convalescence are desirable.

Nursing management

Nursing care aims mainly at relieving symptoms and building up the child's strength and weight. A good general nursing routine is obviously called for as the illness may be a long and tedious one.

The empyema will require to be drained. Chest aspirations may be used at daily intervals. Alternatively a drainage tube may be inserted into the pleural cavity at the site of the empyema and connected to an underwater seal drainage system or into a dressing. The drainage tube may require resiting to be effective. Intensive physiotherapy is important to achieve full expansion of the underlying lung and obliterate the empyema cavity. The nurse should encourage the patient to cough and carry out deep breathing exercises to expand the lung.

Hand in hand with drainage, the empyema is treated by antibiotics given orally, by injection or into the empyema cavity by instillation through the drainage tube.

The patient with empyema looks toxic, his colour is grey and he is apathetic. His appetite is poor and he is often anaemic. The tongue is coated and the temperature may swing at a high level. The diet should be nourishing and appetizing, and extra vitamins may be prescribed. Occupation with suitable play activities will also help to keep the patient happy and at rest.

ASTHMA

Asthma is a respiratory disorder which presents as bronchial spasms, expiratory difficulty, wheezing and a feeling of suffocation. Asthmatic children are very frequently seen in paediatric departments and, during the course of an attack, may present an alarming and pathetic picture. The first attack may occur as early as the first year of life, and occurs more often in boys than girls. Infantile eczema may be replaced by asthma in the older child.

Common causes of asthma

An attack of asthma in the sensitive child may be precipitated by various factors.

Allergic factors

Allergies are thought to be inherited since other members of the family are commonly found to suffer from hay fever, eczema or migraine. In asthma, the allergic factor is most usually inhaled and can usually be traced to the environment. Sensitivity to the house mite, found in dust around the home, is the most important of this group and explains why these children commonly develop their attacks at nights as the house mite finds an ideal dwelling in bedding and mattresses. The house mite lives on shed human skin and prefers humid, warm and dark living conditions. If the child's attacks are noticed to be seasonal, pollen is most likely to be the causative factor. Occasionally, sensitivity to pets occurs and it may be necessary for the pet to be taken care of elsewhere. This is a difficult family decision, but much unnecessary illness can be avoided for the child and this should always be explained to him.

Emotional factors

These can often be observed in the child's relationship with his parents. Very commonly the child is described as being quiet and introspective and is often of above average intelligence.

Infection

Infection may trigger an attack in a child and this is usually of viral origin.

Exercise

Excessive exercise has been implicated in precipitating an attack in the sensitive child.

Nursing management

The nursing care is planned to relieve symptoms, give prescribed treatment and reassure the patient and his parents.

Nursing action	Explanation
Sit the patient up, well supported with pillows. Comfort may be gained by leaning forward on a bed-table covered with a pillow, with an open window nearby.	Respirations are laboured, expiration appearing more difficult than inspiration. There is an audible wheeze.
Oxygen and suction may be required.	The child will appear grey and cyanosed.
Sedation may be required to encourage the child to rest.	The shortage of oxygen and laboured respirations cause the child to be restless and anxious.

Nursing action	**Explanation**
Intravenous infusion may be set up for the administration of anti-spasmodic drugs during the first 24 hours. In persistent attacks corticosteroid therapy may be ordered.	To prevent repeated intravenous injections for administration of drugs.
Parents should be encouraged to stay with the child.	Helps to relieve anxiety.
Diversional play therapy.	Helps to relieve anxiety. Encouragement should be firm and sympathetic.
Sips of cool drink will be soothing. A normal diet will be established fairly quickly.	The breathing difficulties can cause the child to feel nauseated.

General management

Disodium cromoglycate (Intal) or Intal Co. is effective in preventing an asthmatic attack when inhaled through a spinhaler. In the general management of asthma known precipitating factors must be avoided. All pillows and quilts should be Terylene and the mattress should be enclosed in a dust-proof cover. Other beds in the house should be treated in the same way. The mattresses and the house should be vacuumed once a week, with the windows open preferably when the child is out at school. Over-enthusiastic or more frequent vacuuming should be avoided as this only stirs up the dust. Bedroom blinds rather than curtains should be used, and upholstered furniture avoided. The bedroom should be kept warm, dry and well ventilated.

Care should be taken to explain to the parents the nature of asthma, and that the treatment is aimed at reducing the number of attacks. It is important that the parents should not treat the child as an invalid, but encourage him to participate in all school activities. Psychotherapy may be

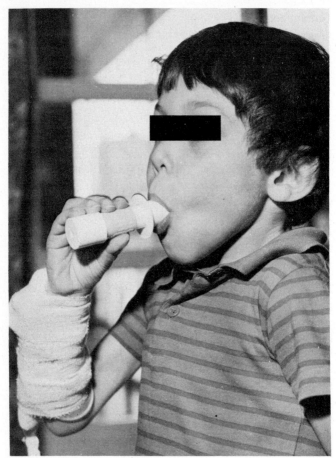

Fig. 25. Asthmatic child using spinhaler.

required for the asthmatic child who is emotionally disturbed. Although the majority of children improve as they
grow older, physiotherapy will be needed throughout childhood in order to prevent the development of a 'pigeon
chest' which in itself leads to repeated chest infections in

later life. Breathing and postural exercises can be taught to the child and his parents in order that they can be carried out regularly in the home.

Investigations

Attempts will be made to identify precipitating causes by means of sensitivity tests. Inspiratory, expiratory and peak flow volumes of air will be estimated.

STATUS ASTHMATICUS

When one attack of acute, spasmodic asthma virtually runs into the next attack, the patient is said to suffer from status asthmaticus.

Treatment and management initially are similar to that in ordinary attacks but, as this state may persist for many hours, exhaustion may be extreme. Relaxation and rest must be achieved by any means available, and this may tax the nurse's ingenuity severely. As so much energy is expended on the act of breathing it is difficult to get the child to take sufficient fluids. Sponging the face and hands, changing and turning the pillows and gentle massage of the patient's scalp with a hair brush can be very soothing. Quiet reassurance by speaking to the child may do much to calm his fears, and hot drinks, given in small amounts as often as possible, help as much as drugs in getting the patient off to sleep.

The child may develop respiratory acidosis, and require intravenous therapy to correct the pH balance and prevent dehydration. Unfortunately, death can no longer be regarded as rare in this condition, and the use of a respirator giving intermittent positive pressure may be life saving.

N.B. One of the reasons for the present increase in deaths of these children whilst in status asthmaticus, is due to the intensive usage of anti-spasmodics before admission to hospital. It is important that an accurate history of the drugs received by the child is known on admission to avoid a lethal dose. The greatest danger comes from aminophylline, which is very toxic in high doses and should not be repeated if there is no response to the initial full dose. Severe asthma may persist throughout life but mild cases may have cleared by the age of 15 years.

BRONCHIOLITIS

Bronchiolitis is most common in infants under 6 months and seldom seen in children over 2 years of age. It tends to occur in epidemics, particularly during the winter. The infecting organism is a virus of which the Respiratory Syncytial Virus (RSV) is the most common. Submucosal inflammation causes obstruction to the bronchioles.

Nursing management

The partial obstruction of the airways in the infant causes difficulty in breathing with the use of accessory muscles of respiration. There is a high respiratory rate of 60–80/min and frequently cyanosis is present. The infant is immediately nursed in a humidified oxygen tent, well supported with pillows.

The rapid pulse and respiratory rates are frequently observed for signs of improvement or deterioration. Difficulty may be encountered identifying the apical heart beat in the acute stages. Precautions are taken to prevent the infant being exerted or becoming cyanosed by reducing the amount of disturbance to as little as possible with planned nursing care.

Antibiotics are seldom prescribed unless a secondary bacterial infection is diagnosed.

Difficulty is encountered in feeding due to the high respiratory rate. Tube feeding of small frequent amounts is often necessary to reduce exertion and maintain nutrition and hydration. The feed may be offered by mouth as the illness subsides.

As the condition improves, tolerance to handling improves. The infant can be picked up and fed as well as being taken out of oxygen for short periods. From being washed in the cot, gradually the infant can be bathed, care being taken not to exhaust the child.

Recovery is slow and the infant is usually discharged during the convalescent period, when the parents feel they are able to manage the child at home and social conditions permit.

The family health visitor should be informed prior to discharge.

Further reading

BALLANTYNE, J. V. & GROVES, J. (1978) *Otolaryngology*. Bristol: Wright.

COOKE, R. W. I. (1979) *A Guide to Ventilator Care of Infants*. London: Vickers Medical.

GREGORY, G. A. (1981) *Respiratory Failure in the Child*. London: Churchill Livingstone.

KUZEMBO, J. A. (1980) *Asthma in Children*. London: Pitman Medical.

NORTHER, J. L. & DOWNS, M. P. (1978) *Hearing in Children*, 2nd edn. Baltimore: Williams & Wilkins.

Office of Health Economics (1976) *Asthma*, No. 57, Series of Papers on current Health Problems. London: Office of Health Economics.

WILLIAMS, H. E. & PHELAN, P. D. (1975) *Respiratory Illness in Children*. London: Blackwell Scientific.

WILLIAMS, H. E. & PHELAN, P. D. (1982) *Respiratory Disease in Children*, 2nd edn. London: Blackwell Scientific.

6 The cardiovascular system

The relationship between temperature, pulse and respirations in children is of great importance and should therefore always be reported together.

The pulse

Owing to the small size of the structures involved, even simple procedures such as taking the pulse or the blood pressure and obtaining a sample of venous blood may present special difficulties in children; the younger the child, the more difficult it may be to feel and count the pulse beat over the radial artery at the wrist as he may resent being touched and may struggle or cry; also, overlying fat may make it hard to feel the pulse and may alter the volume and make assessment difficult. It is often a good plan to try to take the pulse while the patient is sleeping and this is often best done over the temporal artery immediately in front of the ear or in the case of infants over the fontanelle. The pulse should be taken and counted for 1 min. Changes in the rate, volume or rhythm should be reported at once. In certain diseases, for instance in some types of congenital heart disease, the pulse can be plainly seen at the side of the neck, in others it is not palpable in the groin, as it is in normal children. The pulse rate alters as the child grows older and during exercise, excitement or disease. An increased pulse rate (tachycardia) may be associated with pyrexia, the administration of certain drugs and following haemorrhage. An abnormally slow pulse (bradycardia) may be due to raised intercranial pressure. Infection and febrile conditions in infancy are not, however, necessarily accompanied by a rapid pulse as with adults, a fact which must be borne in mind when assessing a child's condition.

Taking the blood pressure

In infants and young children it is difficult to estimate the blood pressure with accuracy. Special narrow cuffs may have to be used. Variations may be considerable even in healthy children, but average systolic readings are likely to be 60–80 mmHg and the diastolic pressure 50–60 mmHg in the first year and 100–110/80 (systolic/diastolic) at 10 years of age, while at rest.

Daily blood pressure readings may be required in certain heart diseases, diseases of the kidney, when increased intracranial pressure is suspected and in the case of patients on steroid therapy. Children are sometimes frightened by the apparatus, and it may be wise to 'reassure' them by taking the teddy-bear's blood pressure first and letting them handle the rubber bulb, making the mercury rise and fall themselves.

Cyanosis

Lack of oxygen in the circulation causes cyanosis more readily in young children than in adults. Central cyanosis is always a serious sign. It should be relieved without delay by the administration of oxygen. It may be particularly marked in respiratory abnormalities of the newborn, congenital heart lesions and in obstructed breathing. Occasionally young children have breath-holding attacks which cause cyanosis. These attacks are often due to behaviour disturbances.

TYPES OF HEART DISEASE IN CHILDHOOD

There are two main types of heart disease in childhood.

1. Congenital malformations of the heart or great blood vessels.
2. Inflammatory lesions in the heart, causing carditis.

Both these will interfere with the action of the heart and lead to heart failure, in an attempt by the heart muscle to compensate for the extra strain placed upon it, thereby becoming weakened and failing to push the necessary amount of blood to the body.

Heart failure in childhood is usually acute. Chronic heart failure develops gradually.

Heart failure

Instant recognition and treatment of developing heart failure in the infant is necessary in order to preserve life. The young baby may collapse in a matter of hours or days, while the older child or adolescent may take weeks before his condition becomes serious.

The most common causes of heart failure are due to:

1. Congenital heart disease.
2. Pulmonary conditions.
3. The anaemias.
4. Carditis.

Nursing management

Nursing action	Explanation
Maintain an upright, supported position.	Prevent abdominal organs pressing on the diaphragm and allow lung expansion.
Administration of oxygen by tent. (Older children by mask.)	The sluggish circulation and reduced cardiac output result in cyanosis, restlessness and irritability.

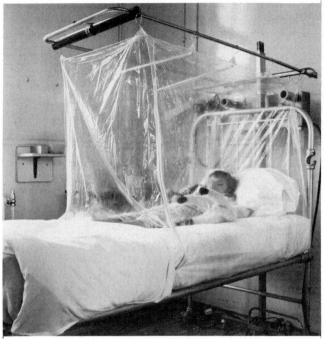

Fig. 26. Child in oxygen tent.

Nursing action	Explanation
Light, loose clothing changed frequently.	Prevent any restriction to breathing.
Regular, frequent recording of body temperature. Mittens and socks to wear on extremities.	Heat lost easily due to sweating and poor circulation. Maintain body heat to reduce metabolic demands.
Frequent observation of pulse and respiratory rate.	Marked tachycardia and abnormal rhythms reported.
Chest physiotherapy.	Persistent cough with thick viscid secretions may block airway.

Nursing action	Explanation
Daily bath and postural position changed every two hours.	Poor peripheral circulation makes these children prone to pressure sores.
Feeds. Give ordinary milk feeds of 150–175 ml/kg body weight/24 h.	Low exercise tolerance and undue exertion should be avoided. Complement feeds by fine nasogastric tube.
Older children require to be tempted with diet. Nursing history will provide likes and dislikes.	To maintain nutrition for normal body requirements.
Frequent mouth care.	Mouth breathing causes drying of mucosa and mouth ulcers.
Mild aperient may be necessary to prevent constipation and prevent abdominal distension.	Difficult defaecation may cause further heart strain.
Record daily weight and fluid intake and output.	Weight gain caused by fluid retention will be detected and patient's general growth observed.

Human milk is relatively low in sodium and if the baby has difficulty in sucking because of low exercise tolerance, the mother should be encouraged to express her breasts. If breast milk is not available SMA may be used.

Drugs

Digoxin acts as a tonic to the heart muscle enabling it to work with greater effect without increasing oxygen consumption. The initial digitalizing dose is larger than the subsequent maintenance dose. The pulse or apex beat should be taken before this drug is administered as undue slowing of the heart beat may occur. Other early toxic symptoms to observe are vomiting, anorexia and irregular or coupling of the heart beat.

Frusemide (Lasix) is a quick-acting diuretic which is

given to stimulate the kidney to excrete water from the body and thereby, salts also. The side-effects of this drug include rapid fluid loss leading to dehydration. Potassium levels in the blood should be frequently assessed and extra potassium given.

Aldactone (spironolactone), a longer-acting diuretic, is occasionally given in divided doses combined with Lasix in patients with severe heart failure.

Morphine is commonly given in order to sedate the patient and reduce the metabolism. This drug also reduces the respiratory rate.

Antibiotics are often prescribed prophylactically as the risk of infection is high in these children.

Play and activity

Children in heart failure tend to be irritable and tire easily, feeling great frustration at not being able to do all the things their friends are able to do.

While doing everything for the child initially, the nurse should encourage him to make small efforts to help himself, e.g. cleaning his teeth, but at the same time she should watch how each small effort affects her patient.

The nurse should choose suitable toys and play activities which do not require too much energy. Parents and the 'play leader' can do much to help keep the child happily occupied and allay restlessness.

The welfare and well-being of the parents may have a great effect on the patient's general condition. The mother's anxiety is easily conveyed unconsciously to the child and will increase his restlessness. If possible the mother should be resident with her child. Parents need to be well-informed about their child's condition and the nurse should be available to listen and support the parents. A social worker should be available to help with particular problems as they arise. The family health visitor and school nurse should be informed before the child is discharged.

Congenital heart disease

Congenital heart disease can be divided as follows:

Acyanotic	*Cyanotic*
Patent ductus arteriosus	Fallot's tetralogy
Coarctation of the aorta	Transposition of the great vessels
Ventricular septal defect	
Atrial septal defect	
Aortic stenosis	
Mitral stenosis	

Patent ductus arteriosus

The ductus arteriosus is necessary to the fetal circulation and failure to close after birth causes oxygenated blood from the aorta (which is under pressure as it leaves the ventricle) to be pumped back into the pulmonary artery where the blood is under low pressure. The flow of blood from the aorta into the pulmonary artery may reach great volumes and the cardiac output is increased. It is not clear why the ductus arteriosus should fail to close in some children although research has shown it to be commonly associated with hypoxia during and after birth. Statistics show that more girls than boys are affected; ratio of 2 : 1.

Growth is often stunted although otherwise there may be no other symptoms. Diagnosis may not be made until the child is 3 or 4 years old, when a heart murmur may be heard on routine medical examination by a doctor. Ligation of the ductus arteriosus is best carried out as soon as the diagnosis is made. The operation is carried out through a left thoracotomy; the heart is not entered. Following successful surgery the patient can expect to lead a normal life.

Coarctation of the aorta

Coarctation means narrowing; in this case narrowing occurs along the course of the aortic arch. The blood supply to the distal part of the aorta is thus reduced, whilst pressure is high in the proximal part—that part of the aorta and the arteries supplied by it which lies between the left ventricle of the heart and the narrowing. The systolic blood pressure in the arm is high, the myocardium hypertrophies in an attempt to increase cardiac output; subsidiary or collateral vessels develop. Pulsation in these vessels can be felt on the chest and back, but the femoral pulse is feeble or absent.

Operation consists of resecting the coarcted area with direct anastomosis. The age that this is performed depends a great deal upon the condition of the individual child and the surgeon, but the surgical correction is recommended before adult life.

In successful cases the prognosis is good. The circulation becomes normal, the blood pressure falls to ordinary levels and the patient is able to lead an active unrestricted life.

Ventricular septal defect

Septal defects between the right and left ventricle vary in size. Small defects (maladie de Roger) are characterized by loud systolic heart murmurs, but the child is often completely asymptomatic and the prognosis is good. No treatment is indicated. It has been reported that some defects close spontaneously.

With large septal defects the situation is different. Due to the higher pressure in the left ventricle, a shunting of blood occurs from the left to right ventricle during systole. This increases the work load of the right ventricle and hypertrophy occurs.

Symptoms may be severe, with marked feeding difficulty, frequent upper respiratory infections and dyspnoea. Growth is impaired. Urgent treatment is required. Operative repair is carried out with the aid of a heart–lung bypass machine. The defect may be repaired by direct closure or with a specially prepared patch, sutured in position. With surgery the prognosis is favourable but the outcome depends upon the amount of resistance which has developed in the pulmonary vascular bed.

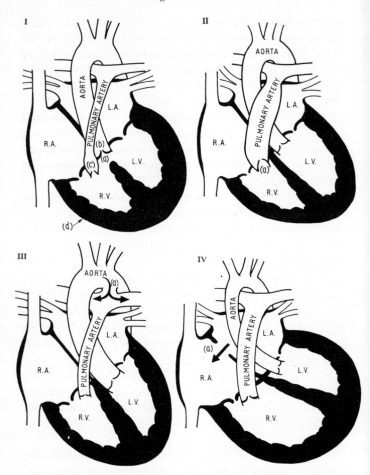

Fig. 27. Congenital malformations of the heart and great vessels. I. Fallot's tetralogy: (a) ventricular septal defect; (b) dextroposition of aorta; (c) pulmonary valvular stenosis; (d) thickened wall of right ventricle. II (a) indicates pulmonary valvular stenosis; III (a) indicates patent ductus arteriosus; IV (a) indicates atrial septal defect.

Atrial septal defects

An atrial septal defect is an abnormal opening in the atrial septum resulting in shunting of blood from the left to right atrium. This produces an increase in the right ventricular output and resultant pulmonary engorgement. The diagnosis is suspected by the presence of a soft blowing systolic murmur in the area of the pulmonary artery that may be found at a routine medical examination.

The child usually appears slight, noticed to tire easily with poor exercise tolerance. Susceptibility to pneumonia and rheumatic fever is increased. Operative repair is possible both by closed and 'open-heart' surgery. Since the prognosis for most of these children is good, the risks of operative repair have to be carefully considered for each individual child.

Aortic stenosis

When a thickening of the aortic semilunar valves occurs it is spoken of as aortic stenosis. The narrowing restricts circulation and causes a lowering of blood pressure in the peripheral arteries; hypertrophy of the left ventricle develops as the heart attempts to overcome the obstruction. Valvotomy is carried out by opening the heart and operating under direct vision.

Fallot's tetralogy

The tetralogy of Fallot varies in severity but is characterized by the combination of four defects.

1. Pulmonary stenosis.
2. Ventricular septal defect.
3. Over-riding aorta.
4. Hypertrophy of the right ventricle.

As a result some of the right ventricular output goes to the aorta. Cyanosis in varying degrees occurs, which is most marked on exertion. It is the most common defect causing cyanosis in patients surviving beyond 2 years of age.

Attacks of paroxysmal dyspnoea may occur in children with Fallot's tetralogy, especially before the age of 2 years. The child becomes distressed with deep cyanosis and air hunger which may be followed by loss of consciousness and convulsions. The child should be placed in the knee-chest position to increase cardiac efficiency and oxygen should be given if available. Older children learn amazingly well to adapt their activities, so that during play they take frequent rest pauses and adopt the characteristic squatting position.

Correction of this anomaly is a major procedure in which the cardiac bypass machine is used. The best age for such surgery depends upon the individual patient.

Transposition of the great vessels

In this anomaly the aorta arises from the right ventricle instead of the left ventricle and the pulmonary artery from the left ventricle. Unless surgical treatment can be given, death usually takes place within a few weeks. A palliative procedure has been developed: *Rashkind balloon atrial septostomy* which creates an atrial septal defect sufficient to maintain similar right and left atrial pressures. This procedure is carried out under a local anaesthetic at cardiac catheterization, before the age of 2 months whilst the septum is reasonably supple. A surgical septostomy through a thoracotomy is performed in the older infant and child—Blalock–Hanlon operation.

The Mustard Procedure has been devised to bring about an internal redirection of blood flow in order that deoxygenated blood will flow into the pulmonary artery. This major surgery is carried out very selectively with the use of the cardiac bypass machine usually after the age of 6 months. The colour change in the child is most dramatic.

He often feels for the first time that he can play without having to sit down at the slightest exertion. The correction may not be adequate to maintain a reasonable level of activity when the child is older.

Cardiac surgery

The recent advances in cardiac surgery are related to improved diagnostic scanning techniques. This enables the cardiothoracic team to prepare the child and his parents for surgery to be performed, this frequently involves the use of intensive post-operative care and its consequent technology. In order to give comfort and support to their child parents should always be offered residential accommodation.

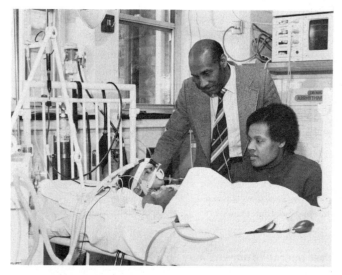

Fig. 28. Child receiving intensive care with anxious parents.

Pre-operative nursing management

Nursing action

1. The child is admitted 3–4 days before operation; introduce parents and child to other families in the ward.

2. The surgeon should interview the parents before they sign the operation consent form.

3. Explanation, according to age, should be given to the child. Opportunities for equipment to be used post-operatively to be demonstrated and played with as part of the play experience in the ward.

4. Investigations will include blood taking for cross-matching, bleeding and clotting times, haemoglobin and electrolyte estimations. Chest X-ray and electrocardiographs and electro-encephalograms.

5. Recordings of blood pressure, temperature, pulse and respirations.

6. Height and weight recorded.

7. With the physiotherapist teach the child breathing exercises for lung expansion.

Explanation

To allow time for physical examination and assessment to take place and for the exploration of the new surroundings for the child and his parents.

To explain the procedure and discuss operative risks involved.

To offset anxiety when recovering from anaesthetic.

To ensure that the child is fit for operation and to ensure the child's safety at operation and post-operatively.

If there is any evidence of infection the operation will be postponed.

For estimation of drug dosage and fluid replacement.

To enable the child to cooperate post-operatively.

Post-operative nursing management

1. For the first 24 hours nursed flat with a wooden board beneath the mattress.

In case of need for emergency resuscitation purposes.

Nursing action	**Explanation**
2. An individual nurse at the child's bedside.	To closely observe for detailed changes in the child's condition.
3. Quarter-hourly observation and recording of all vital signs. Any marked changes or trends are reported immediately.	Early warning indications of impending change, e.g. haemorrhage, shock, etc.
4. Intravenous fluid/blood transfusions should run according to instructions.	To replace blood loss and maintain hydration.
5. Urinary catheter released every hour and recorded on fluid balance chart.	Indication of return of renal functioning.
6. Chest drains are observed for patency and drainage which is measured and recorded.	Indicates returning lung expansion or haemorrhage.
7. Post-operative analgesia, e.g. pethidine or Omnopon.	Reduces shock and pain.
8. Chest physiotherapy and passive limb exercises given. Child turned 2-hourly.	To encourage lung expansion, prevent chest infection and to prevent general circulatory complications.
9. Parents should see their child immediately post-operatively. Reinforce pre-operative explanations of care.	Best method of relieving anxiety of the child and his parents.
10. Nasogastric tube on free drainage and measurement. Nil by mouth.	Indication of return of normal intestinal peristalsis.
11. Frequent mouth care.	To avoid soreness of the mouth and promote comfort.

After 24 hours

1. Removal of urinary catheter.	If kidney function is satisfactory.

Nursing action	**Explanation**
2. Gradually sit child up then slowly mobilize to sit in a chair.	To prevent vascular and chest complications.
3. Deep breathing exercises continued.	To fully expand lungs.
4. Intercostal chest drains are removed after a satisfactory chest X-ray.	Lungs are usually fully expanded 24–48 h post-operatively.
5. Small amounts of clear fluids offered orally and when these are tolerated the nasogastric tube is removed. Light diet gradually introduced.	Gastrointestinal function gradually returns to normal.
6. Increasing active play occupation provided.	Will encourage return to normal activities.
7. Glycerin suppository may be necessary to aid bowel action.	
8. Sutures usually removed after a week.	

If the recovery period continues uneventfully the child is discharged home about the 10th day post-operatively. Parents should be advised as to the best routine to follow at home for the needs of their child. The child initially should be encouraged to rest in the afternoons, gradually doing more and more. After relief of a serious cardiac disability babies often find themselves enjoying their feeds for the first time. They are inclined to take them greedily, demanding more than is offered. The temptation to overfeed must be resisted to avoid overdistension and pressure on the diaphragm.

A follow-up appointment for all patients to visit out-patients is given usually 4–6 weeks after discharge. It is most rewarding for the nurse to see her patients when they come back looking very well, able to play more games with their friends and also to notice the relief of tension and anxiety in the family.

Assisted ventilation

The aim of assisted ventilation is to maintain gas exchange in the lungs (see p. 52). The child is attached to the ventilator by a tracheal tube.

Nursing management

Nursing action	Explanation
Aspiration of the tracheal tube at least 2-hourly or when secretions can be heard rattling in the tube.	To maintain a patent airway.
Carried out gently and swiftly.	The ventilator is temporarily disconnected to allow aspiration to be carried out.
Care of the tube. Secure tube with tapes.	To avoid dislodging the tube.
Support ventilator tubing weight.	To prevent weight pulling tube out.
Observation of patient. Record of the patient's pulse, respirations and temperature is kept. Colour observed.	Monitor change in condition.
Observation of ventilator. Rate of ventilator, inspiratory and expiratory flow, tidal volume and flow of gases are recorded.	To identify any change in patient or machine.
Humidification flow is observed and condensation in tubing removed.	All children require humidified gases to be administered.
Administration of respiratory depressant drugs.	To maintain syncronization with the ventilator.
Child should never be left unattended.	In case child becomes disconnected from machine.
Talk to the child. Communicate by writing or drawing. Tell stories, play records, etc.	Although the child cannot respond by talking he will enjoy the stimulation which will help to allay anxiety.

Weaning the child from the machine

Either the child can be encouraged to breathe spontaneously during increasing lengths of time of disconnection from the ventilator, or the trigger mechanism is adjusted to encourage the child to greater effort in establishing the onset of inspiration.

Hypothermia

The ability of certain organs of the body to remain undamaged if deprived of oxygen at normal temperature is known to vary and it is known that the brain tissues are the first to suffer, the maximum period of deprivation for the brain being 4 min without causing irreparable damage. By cooling the body to temperatures as low as 12°–15°C (53°–60°F) the metabolism is slowed down and therefore the oxygen requirements reduced. Operations involving a temporary interruption of circulation can therefore be undertaken while the patient is in a state comparable to that of a hibernating animal.

Cooling of the body can be achieved by the use of ice packs, by immersion in cooled water or by allowing the blood to flow through a cannula and tubing from the superior vena cava to a refrigerating circuit and pumping it back into the circulation via the inferior vena cava.

Care of intercostal drainage

Following intrathoracic surgery one or two tubes are stitched into position to allow fluid and air to escape from the pleural space. The drainage tube connects to a drainage bottle either containing a measured amount of water or suitable disinfectant or in some cases a 'Redivac' sealed bottle. This forms an air-tight seal.

Expansion of the chest on inspiration increases the intrapleural vacuum and as fluid and air drains out the lungs re-expand. Drainage must be carefully measured, and fluctuations in the tube noted. The tubes should be 'milked' at frequent intervals to prevent blockage of the tube lumen.

When the lungs are fully expanded drainage ceases; following X-ray confirmation of this, the tube is removed under aseptic conditions carefully sealing the tube entry point with sterile vaseline on a gauze dressing to prevent air entry.

The tube leading to the drainage bottle must be clipped off securely when changing the bottle and it must never be raised above the level of the patient, or air and fluid may be sucked back into the plural space.

Special diagnostic procedures

Angiography

Radio-opaque dye is injected into the venous circulation. Serial radiographs or cine-recording follows the passage of the dye through the heart, outlining abnormal shunts or any obstruction. This procedure is commonly combined with cardiac catheterization.

Cardiac catheterization

Under deep sedation an opaque catheter is inserted by way of a vein, commonly one of the femoral veins, into the superior vena cava, the right atrium, right ventricle and pulmonary artery. Pressures and oxygen saturations are measured repeatedly during the procedure revealing a great deal of information about the function of the heart. The use of serial radiographs and/or cine-recording enables the doctor to follow the progress of the catheter.

Catheterization of the left side of the heart in the absence of any shunt is much more difficult and must be performed either through the aorta or by perforation of the atrial septum within the heart as in Rashkind's procedure.

Cardiac catheterization is not without risk. This procedure should be carried out in specialist paediatric centres. After the procedure the child should be carefully observed for blood loss from the site of the venous incision, and resultant shock. Nursing care is aimed at keeping the child quiet and rested. Oxygen and humidity being given if necessary. Providing all observations are satisfactory the child may be up and about in 24–48 h. The wound should be kept dry and the sutures removed about the seventh day.

Haematocrit

The haematocrit or packed cell volume becomes elevated with cyanosis and is accompanied by an increased viscosity of the blood. This increased viscosity heightens the patient's susceptibility to cerebral thrombosis.

Echocardiogram

This non-invasive technique demonstrates the outline and structures of the heart. When demonstrated upon a television screen the structures are in 3-dimension, the single plate is flat. This technique is new and requires skilled interpreters of the pictures obtained. The benefit of its use is that the child is not subjected to invasive diagnostic procedures. The child is required to remain still during the procedure and may require sedation to do this.

Inflammatory heart diseases

Although endocarditis, myocarditis and pericarditis are separate entities, any one of them is bound to affect all parts of the heart as the various structures are intimately connected.

Inflammation may be caused by toxins reaching the heart as in pneumonia, influenza, general septicaemia and especially diphtheria, and the result may be heart failure. Alternatively the heart may be affected by bacterial invasion, e.g. bacterial endocarditis. Inflammatory heart disease is one of the possible complications of rheumatic fever and chorea. Permanent cardiac damage may result.

Bacterial endocarditis

Bacterial endocarditis is an acute or more commonly a sub-acute infection of the endocardium and this condition often follows throat, dental or middle ear infections caused by *Streptococcus viridans*. Bacterial endocarditis usually arises as a complication of congenital or rheumatic heart disease. It is rare in childhood.

The symptoms are similar to those of rheumatic carditis but the child is extremely toxic. He looks seriously ill, the eyes are sunken and surrounded by deep shadows and though he seems weary he tosses about restlessly. Pulse and respiration rates are increased and the temperature may rise to 40°C (104°F) or more. The skin becomes dry, the urinary output is diminished, the tongue is furred, the lips dry and inclined to crack. Petechial spots may appear on the skin.

The child will be nursed in a similar manner as that described for a child with cardiac failure.

Drug therapy is directed towards overcoming the infections by giving large doses of the appropriate antibiotic, usually one of the penicillins. In very severe cases this may be given intravenously. Steroids are prescribed because of their anti-inflammatory effect and to minimize the production of scar tissue.

Recovery may be complete but the illness and period of convalescence may extend over many months. A careful follow-up by the paediatrician must be maintained over several years.

Complications

1. Embolism as a result of breakdown from the septic valves.

2. Permanent damage to the valves requiring operation at a later date.

Further reading

GRAHAM, G. (1980) *Heart Disease in Infants and Children*. London: Edward Arnold.

JORDON, S. C. & SCOTT, O. (1981) *Heart Disease in Paediatrics*, 2nd edn. London: Butterworth.

LEVIN, D. L. (1979) *A Practical Guide to Paediatric Intensive Care*. St. Louis: C. V. Mosby.

Nursing Times (1980) *Intensive Care of the Newborn*. London: Macmillan Journals.

THOMPSON, D. R. (1982) *Cardiac Nursing*. London: Baillière Tindall.

7 Rheumatic and collagen disorders

All the diseases described in this chapter are thought to be due to a hypersensitivity or an autoimmunity reaction. In persons affected by any of these conditions, the normal immune reaction is replaced by an abnormal sensitivity to infection or a definite destructive reaction within the body. In addition to the conditions described in this chapter, the following diseases are sometimes included in this broad group:

Anaphylactoid purpura (see p. 182).

Idiopathic and symptomatic thrombocytopenic purpuras (see p. 193).

Nephritis, nephrosis (see pp. 349 and 353).

Ulcerative colitis.

ACUTE RHEUMATIC FEVER AND RHEUMATIC CARDITIS

In acute rheumatic fever there is commonly a history of a sore throat or tonsillitis 2 or 3 weeks before the onset of symptoms.

Streptococcus pyogenes is usually the causative organism, but this is not always present on culture when a throat swab is taken. The infection may have been overcome although the streptococcal toxin has set up an autoimmune reaction in the body.

The child suffering from acute rheumatic fever often has a moderate pyrexia, a raised pulse rate and general toxic signs such as headache, vomiting, furred tongue, sweating and constipation. The child may complain of polyarthritis and the severe pain may affect one joint one day and others the next. Occasionally a faint, slightly pink rash appears on the trunk and this may recur intermittently (erythema marginatum). Rheumatic nodules are sometimes found over the elbows, shins, knuckles, knees, occiput and spine. These nodules are usually a sign that the illness is taking a serious course and they are rarely found unless the heart has become affected.

Nursing management

The child requires exertion to be reduced to a minimum. Complete rest is enforced, the child doing as little for himself and being nursed in a recumbent position. The nurse will have to explain this if the child is old enough and capable of cooperation. Occasionally the child may have to be fed, but some paediatricians feel that, provided the child is well supported with pillows, to feed himself causes the minimal amount of strain. Two nurses will be required for giving a bedpan without sitting the patient up.

The child requires to be nursed in a warm, quiet corner or room where there is minimal danger of other children or passers-by knocking the bed. Even a slight vibration may cause the child to cry out in pain. A firm mattress should be used and the weight of the bedclothes relieved with a bedcradle. The painful joints may be relieved by support with a small pillow, and pads of warm cotton wool may give comfort.

The nurse can use her nursing skill and imagination in many ways to relieve pain and boredom and to make the irksome rest and the difficulties of taking food in a recumbent position as bearable as possible. The use of plastic straws eases the drinking problem. Appropriate play activities will need to be planned which enlist the help of the child's visitors. Radio and television help to allay boredom and keep activity to a minimum.

The temperature, pulse and respiration are observed every 4 hours. The pulse should be noted, particularly for quality and rhythm as well as rate. The sleeping pulse should be recorded every 3 hours to detect early signs of carditis. A fluid balance chart is kept and an imbalance in the intake and output may be an early sign of cardiac failure. Provided bed scales are available the child's weekly weight should be checked.

Progress is monitored by the erythrocyte sedimentation rate together with sleeping pulse recordings. A gradual increase in exercise is allowed as the clinical picture improves. If general symptoms persist and cardiac symptoms persist or occur, rheumatic carditis may have followed the attack of acute rheumatism.

Endocarditis, with some involvement of the myocardium, is the most common manifestation and the pathology is similar to that of endocarditis in the adult. The lesions resulting from the inflammatory process are scarring and growth of vegetation around the cardiac valves causing permanent damage such as heart failure, mitral stenosis, aortic valve incompetence and pericarditis. The child with rheumatic carditis will be in bed for a number of weeks and require continuing total nursing care during this time.

Drug therapy

Salicylates are the specific drugs for the treatment of acute rheumatic conditions. Usually 0.6 g four times a day is given in the form of Disprin or Solprin. Relief from pain may be very rapid. Signs of intolerance should always be watched for and reported at once. These include nausea, tinnitus, vomiting, deafness, albuminuria, a discrete erythematous, sighing respirations and purpura.

Steroids are used to prevent cardiac damage. They are used with caution and are found to be particularly valuable in severe cases of acute rheumatic fever with carditis.

Prophylactic antibiotics against recurrent streptococcal infections is sometimes prescribed and usually carried on for a period of five years or until the child leaves school, whichever is the longer.

Digoxin may be ordered if there is any cardiac incompetence due to carditis, together with frusemide (Lasix) if oedema presents.

CHOREA (SYNDENHAM'S CHOREA, 'ST. VITUS' DANCE')

Chorea is characterized by involuntary, uncoordinated and purposeless movements. The onset is often insidious but emotional factors do appear to play a part in starting the disease. The child becomes fidgety, frequently dropping things and his handwriting deteriorates. Emotionally the child becomes labile. The movements cease during sleep.

Nursing management

Cot sides should be used to prevent the child falling out of bed and in severe cases these may need to be padded to prevent injury. The child may be nursed with the aid of sheepskins and bedcradles to prevent friction sores. Sudden noises and lights should be avoided and all excitement kept from the patient. Drinking and feeding may present difficulties due to the continuous movements, and it may be necessary to resort to nasogastric tube feeding. The mouth should be given special attention as the child frequently bites his tongue, lips or cheeks and ulceration easily occurs. Axillary temperature must be taken to prevent accidents, and a sleeping pulse rate recorded.

Complete recovery may be expected after several weeks but there is a tendency for recurrence and the danger of cardiac involvement is considerable.

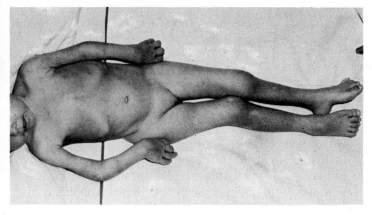

Fig. 29. Still's disease. Note deformities of joints.

RHEUMATOID ARTHRITIS
(STILL'S DISEASE)

Still's disease (Fig. 29) is an inflammatory condition of the joints, similar to the more common, crippling condition known as rheumatoid arthritis in adults. Although not common in childhood, Still's disease is of interest to the paediatric nurse because of the characteristic manifestations and the careful nursing called for in this disease.

Still's disease most commonly starts between the age of 18 months and 6 years and the earlier the onset the less favourable the prognosis. The cause remains unknown.

Signs and symptoms

The first manifestation of the disease may be a single swollen joint (often the knee). A carefully taken history may reveal recurrent complaints of a stiff neck or stiffness in other joints. Occasionally the onset is acute and may easily be mistaken for acute rheumatic fever. The child is feverish and complains of general malaise. Pain and swelling of the joints may be both acute and severe. More often, however, the disease develops gradually. The usually bright child becomes listless, miserable and pale. Loss of appetite soon causes him to lose weight and he fails to make general progress. He has a high, swinging temperature, the skin is moist and clammy and the blood sedimentation rate is raised (50–100 mm in one hour) and the Rose Waaler test may be positive. The haemoglobin level falls and there may be a mild degree of tachycardia. On examination, sub-cutaneous nodules may be found although more rarely than in rheumatic fever. As the illness progresses the joints become more painful and swollen and the overlying skin looks white and shiny, though at the same time it may be hot to the touch. Periarticular swelling and wasting gradually cause the fingers to take on a spindle-shaped appearance.

As a rule the fingers, wrists, elbows and knees, feet and cervical spine are affected most and the swellings and deformity occur symmetrically. Despite marked swellings in the acute stages, the joints are not always permanently damaged, though fibrous ankylosis is very often the cause of extensive crippling and may necessitate corrective orthopaedic surgery. Osteoporosis may be considerable and may be the cause of pathological fractures. Occasionally a fine erythematous rash appears and may not fade for many weeks. Both the peripheral lymphatic glands and the spleen may be enlarged. Pericarditis is an occasional complication.

Treatment

In the acute stage this aims at resting both the patient and the affected part, and splints are applied to avoid deformity. The child should be nursed in a well-ventilated room and the bed should be protected from any jarring movement. Whenever possible he should be carried onto a balcony or into the garden but draughts and colds should be avoided. The bedclothes should be light and bedcradles should be used. Sandbags, small pillows and foot rests, and light plaster of Paris splints help to make the patient more comfortable and may prevent deformities. Even in the acute stages, physiotherapy should ensure movement through the whole range at least once daily. Movement may be made easier by heat therapy prior to physiotherapy and this can be achieved by the use of radiant heat, wax baths or infra-red ray treatment, but it should be remembered that the child must not be left even for a short time during such treatment.

The diet should be attractive and nutritious and should contain adequate amounts of vitamins. Fresh fruit is wholesome and may help to prevent constipation. Poor general health and immobility make careful attention to all pressure areas important. Children with Still's disease are inclined to become overanxious and introspective, and schooling and adequate occupation should be provided to keep up the child's morale and interest. At the same time occupational therapy will help to keep the affected joints moving.

Drug therapy

Salicylates which abolish pain and fever in acute rheumatism are also effective in Still's disease. The possibility of salicylate intestinal bleeding must be kept in mind, but Disprin and other analgesics may relieve pain. Iron is given to combat anaemia and occasionally a small blood transfusion may help to build up the child's health generally, as well as raising the haemoglobin level. Steroids are used with some success, but the side-effects which occur, and the need to keep up the steroid therapy, limit their usefulness. If only one or two joints are affected, intra-articular hydrocortisone may be of value. However, if this treatment is used for weight-bearing joints, caution must be observed lest the relief of symptoms leads to excessive use of the joint thus causing further damage.

Prognosis

Inadequate or late treatment may lead to complications which include general ill health, retarded growth, deformities and blindness from iridocyclitis. About half the children suffering from Still's disease and treated within a year of onset, may be expected to have no residual joint lesions 5 years later; the disease may, in others, burn itself out over a period of 1–2 years.

OTHER COLLAGEN DISEASES

Sometimes a hypersensitivity or autoimmune reaction affects the connective tissue, and in that case one of five rare diseases, grouped together as collagen diseases, may occur. These diseases are briefly described below. They may have a poor prognosis in spite of treatment with steroids and death is often caused by renal failure. The serum proteins are abnormal and the erythrocyte sedimentation rate is raised.

Henoch-Schönlein's syndrome (anaphylactoid purpura)

Henoch-Schönlein's purpura, which is one of the collagen diseases, is seen fairly commonly in childhood, but rarely before the age of 3 years. The small purpuric haemorrhages seen on the skin are at first of a purple colour but later they turn a dusky red and still later, brown, until they gradually disappear. A faint urticarial rash is usually present. The areas most commonly involved are the legs, the back of the elbows and arms, the lumbar region and buttocks. Any pressure, such as sitting on a bedpan, may cause localized purpuric spots. If the haemorrhages involve the intestinal tract, there may be severe abdominal pain of a colicky nature which may last for several hours. This may be followed by the passage of bright blood or a melaena stool. The child may be shocked and occasionally an intussusception may complicate the picture. For that reason there is a certain danger in giving drugs such as pethidine to relieve pain, as this may mask symptoms which should urgently be recognized. The Henoch-Schönlein syndrome may also involve the large joints causing pain and swelling although there is no actual haemorrhage into the joint itself. As different joints become involved, pain flits from one site to another but it never leaves permanent damage or stiffness.

Often no specific treatment is considered necessary and with bed rest the child gradually improves and the rash fades after about 2 or 3 weeks. Steroids may, however, be given if the erythrocyte sedimentation rate is high or if there is albuminuria. There is a tendency for recurrence.

Complications

Complications include nephritis and intussusception, which are dealt with in the usual way.

Nursing management

Nursing care is symptomatic. Relief of pain for the affected joints may be given by applying pads of warmed cotton wool and in cases of severe abdominal pain a well-protected hot water bottle might be used with special permission from the ward sister. Gentle massage may bring some comfort. A painful limb may be elevated on a small pillow and a bedcradle should be used to take the weight of the bedclothes. Pressure from the rim of a bedpan should be excluded by padding it with an air ring or by using a rubber pan.

Polyarteritis nodosa (periarteritis nodosa)

Polyarteritis nodosa is an acute inflammation of the small arterioles, with aneurysm formation which can sometimes be quite easily felt as nodules under the skin. The damage to the arterioles may lead to thrombosis and to haemorrhage. The main signs and symptoms are fever, tachycardia, joint and muscle pains and proteinuria which may progress to renal failure. There is hypertension and a polymorphonuclear leucocytosis, and anaemia is common. Temporal arteritis may cause severe headaches and possibly cerebral haemorrhage. Renal and muscle biopsy will confirm the diagnosis.

Dermatomyositis

Dermatomyositis has an insidious onset. Muscle, skin and subcutaneous tissues become inflamed. The muscles are stiff, tender and swollen and become weak with atrophy, contractions and fibrosis. The heart muscle may be affected, causing myocarditis and tachycardia. There is a typical, violet-coloured rash on cheeks and eyelids, circumoral pallor, and an erythematous and sometimes urticarial rash on trunk, limbs and knuckles. The subcutaneous tissues become inelastic and there is a low grade pyrexia and progressive disability which may include muscles of respiration, speech and swallowing. The urinary creatinine levels are greatly elevated in the acute phase, and muscle biopsy and electromyogram confirm the diagnosis. The condition may become chronic with signs similar to scleroderma, but in spite of steroid therapy acute cases may die of cardiac or renal failure or intercurrent infections.

Lupus erythematosus

The disseminated form of lupus erythematosus is rare in childhood, and has an even worse prognosis than in later life. The most characteristic lesion is a purplish-red, raised and indurated 'butterfly' rash over the cheeks and nose. All the mesenchymal tissues are affected, leading to hypertension, anaemia, pyrexia, painful swelling of joints, enlargement of liver and spleen, pleurisy, endocarditis, proteinuria and renal lesions. The bone marrow is depressed, causing leucopenia, and the blood sedimentation rate is very high. Atypical antibodies from the autoimmune reaction—lupus erythematosus (LE) cells—can be seen in blood tests and are specially diagnostic. Treatment is with prednisone 1–2 mg/kg/day initially, but other immunosuppressive agents such as azathioprine 2–5 mg/kg/day may be given.

Further reading

ANSELL, B. M. (1980) *Rheumatic Disorders in Childhood*. London: Butterworth.

BRUNNER, L. S. & SUDDARTH, D. S. (1981) *The Lippincott Manual of Paediatric Nursing*. London: Harper & Row.

WHALEY, L. F. & WONG, D. L. (1979) *Nursing Care of Infants and Children*. St. Louis: C. V. Mosby.

WILLIAMS, G. F. (1981) *Children with Chronic Arthritis*. Massachusetts: P.S.G. Publishing.

8 Haematological disorders

Anaemia, the most common disorder of the blood in childhood, is due to a reduction in the quality or the quantity of red blood cells (erythrocytes), and reduces the oxygen carrying power of the blood. Apart from a decrease in the number of red blood cells or the quantity of haemoglobin present, alterations in the shape and size of these cells may also occur.

Classification of anaemias

Deficiency anaemias
Decreased blood formation due to:
 (a) Too few red blood cells.
 (b) Too little haemoglobin in red cells.

Haemolytic anaemias
Increased haemolysis (blood destruction) due to:
 (a) Production of abnormal red blood cells.
 (b) Abnormal destruction of red blood cells.

Haemorrhagic anaemias
Due to blood loss, acute or chronic.

Clinical picture of anaemia
When the onset is insidious mother often first notices the child to be listless, apathetic and tiring more easily than his playmates. The young baby often refuses feeds or may not

complete them. The older child sometimes complains of headaches, giddiness and blurred vision. In the younger child pica (dirt eating) may be observed, this usually stops once the cause of the anaemia has been treated.

Mother will notice that the child is difficult over eating, refusing previously well-liked foods. Episodes of sepsis and upper respiratory tract infections are very common, often necessitating frequent absence from school. In severe cases, dyspnoea and some puffiness or oedema of the lower limbs may be present. On physical examination the doctor may hear a cardiac murmur.

Some children with anaemia appear pale, but this is deceptive as red cheeks or a dark skin may hide severe anaemia. The colour of the conjunctivae or of the mucous membrane are more important to observe as these will appear pale in the anaemic child.

When anaemia develops rapidly, e.g. after haemorrhage, the child will appear limp and breathless with a marked tachycardia within a very short time.

Whenever anaemia is suspected it is important that a specimen of blood is obtained before treatment is commenced in order that the primary cause of the anaemia be detected as quickly as possible.

DEFICIENCY ANAEMIAS

Hypoplastic and aplastic anaemia

Failure of the bone marrow to manufacture erythrocytes completely is called *aplastic anaemia* but fortunately this is rare. *Hypoplastic anaemia* or underproduction of erythrocytes may occur. These conditions may be caused by certain drugs, e.g. chloramphenicol, but often the cause is unknown. Diagnosis is established by bone marrow puncture. The white cells and platelets are usually also reduced, so that these children suffer from infections and bleeding as well as anaemia.

Treatment consists of giving whole blood or packed cell transfusions in order to provide the mature red cells. These transfusions need to be given repeatedly and one day admissions to hospital will be necessary. The child should be admitted to the same ward each time so that he returns to people and surroundings who are familiar to him and so eventually comes to accept this process as part of his normal routine. Steroids may be given and occasionally the bone marrow recovers spontaneously, but the disease is commonly fatal.

NUTRITIONAL DEFICIENCY ANAEMIA

Iron deficiency

Iron deficiency is the most common of the nutritional deficiency anaemias and indeed of all the childhood anaemias. Iron is essential for the production of haemoglobin and deficiency may be due to:

1. Insufficient iron in the diet.
2. To prematurity, multiple births or maternal anaemia before birth of the baby.
3. Failure to absorb iron in the gastrointestinal tract following neonatal surgery, or with malabsorption syndromes, e.g. coeliac disease.

Iron deficiency anaemia is most common in those infants fed on a milk-only diet after the age of 4–5 months, when all the reserves of iron stored in the liver have been used up. Infants are particularly at risk for the development of this condition as the stores of iron in the liver are built up during the last months of pregnancy. The onset is gradual. Increased susceptibility to infection is often the first indication that anaemia may be present.

In later childhood this anaemia follows infection, especially of the gastrointestinal tract. Intestinal parasites combined with infection and a poor diet will add to the iron deficiency.

Folic acid and vitamin B_{12} deficiency

Folic acid and vitamin B_{12} are essential for the synthesis of nucleoproteins for the maturation of red blood cells. A deficiency of these constituents results in the red blood cells being immature and larger than normal (megaloblastic).

Management

Prophylactic addition of iron to all pre-term infants from the age of 1 month.

Mixed feeding to all babies is introduced from about the age of 4 months. Some paediatricians advocate iron supplements from the age of 12–16 weeks until mixed feeding is fully established. As with other medicines this should never be added to the milk feed but given separately.

Children often accept iron medicines more readily than they do pills. They can be given either through a straw or from a spoon. Older children should be encouraged to brush their teeth after taking the medicine, as in some cases they may produce some discoloration of the teeth. For all ages it is best to give the prescribed preparation before a meal.

As well as giving iron supplements the appetite should be stimulated with an attractive, well-balanced diet rich in iron-containing foods:

| Eggs | Liver | Chocolate | Dried fruits |
| Meat | Fish | Fruit | Wholemeal bread |

It is important that adequate amounts of vitamin C, copper, folic acid and vitamin B are also present in the diet as these are also essential for the development of mature red blood cells.

The nurse should remember that anaemic children tire more easily than their friends, and will often need a rest during the day or a quiet play period instead of joining in more boisterous games.

In severe cases a blood transfusion may be necessary to replace the missing haemoglobin and stimulate the bone marrow. Intramuscular iron is not usually prescribed for children but intravenous iron may be given at the commencement of treatment for severe anaemia.

When anaemia is associated with malabsorption syndrome the underlying cause must be treated with the addition of vitamin and iron supplements to the diet.

HAEMOLYTIC ANAEMIAS

Haemolytic anaemias are due to excessive and rapid breakdown of red blood cells, and patients may become jaundiced as the haemoglobin released from the broken-down cells is converted into the bile pigment, bilirubin. Treatment consists of repeated blood transfusions. The most important haemolytic anaemia in childhood is haemolytic disease of the newborn which is considered on p. 57.

Acute haemolytic anaemia

Acute haemolytic anaemia is characterized by a rapid destruction of red blood cells, so that haemoglobin and red blood cells fall dramatically in a very short time. The spleen is enlarged, petechial haemorrhages may occur in the skin, mild pyrexia may be present and the child is listless, fractious and acutely ill. Vomiting and diarrhoea may aggravate the condition. The illness is usually cured by blood transfusion, but may continue as a chronic acquired haemolytic anaemia which needs to be controlled by the use of steroids.

This disease may be caused by drugs, sulphonamides and antimalarial agents in susceptible people who can be shown to have a deficiency of the enzyme G6PD (glucose-6-phosphate dehydrogenase) in their red blood cells. This deficiency is inherited as a sex-linked trait, and is most common in people of negro descent, Italians, Greeks, Oriental Jews and Arabs.

Acholuric jaundice (hereditary spherocytosis)

The cause of this haemolytic anaemia is the unusual fragility of the red blood cells resulting in rapid haemolysis producing jaundice. The spleen is enlarged and firm. Latent periods and exacerbations occur. Crises are often caused by infections and at such times the jaundice deepens, the child may complain of severe abdominal pain, his general condition is poor and may even give rise to anxiety.

Blood transfusion may be needed during a crisis, otherwise a good diet with therapeutic amounts of iron as indicated by the haemoglobin level and prompt treatment of any infection is needed. Splenectomy may be necessary but should only be performed when the child is free from infection and able to tolerate operation. Removal of the spleen produces a clinical cure and prevents the risk of traumatic injury to the enlarged spleen.

Thalassaemia

Thalassaemia (or Cooley's haemolytic anaemia) occurs in families of Mediterranean origin. The cause is the failure of change from fetal haemoglobin to the more mature adult form. Severity of the disease is determined by inheritance.

In the homozygous child (inherited from both parents) anaemia is very severe, marked by extreme fatigue and apathy; repeated infections occur. The child will be noticed to be 'pot-bellied' due to the enlarged liver and spleen and growth is stunted.

Treatment consists of frequent fresh blood transfusions with long-term desferrioxamine therapy to minimize the accumulation of iron in the tissues (haemosiderosis). Folic acid 5 mg daily should also be given. The prognosis is poor due to heart or liver failure.

Sickle cell anaemia

Sickle cell anaemia is common amongst black races. An abnormal form of haemoglobin is present in this disease, with the beta chain amino acid sequence being altered. During low oxygen concentration these abnormal red cells distort and become 'sickle' shaped. This haemoglobin-opathy results in excess haemolysis and may occur in two forms. Inheritance of the recessive gene from both parents (homozygous) results in severe anaemia and jaundice, with repeated attacks of pain and fever. The pain is caused by the effect of sickled cells becoming impacted in capillaries where oxygen tension is low, such as intestine, joints and kidneys. The abnormal shaped cell is liable to destruction by the spleen. Anaemia results from the rate of destruction of red cells exceeding the rate of production. Treatment is aimed at allowing the child to lead as normal a life as possible and protect against possible infection. Repeated transfusions of packed blood cells will be necessary in order to maintain the level of haemoglobin.

The minor form of sickle cell disease (heterozygous) may go undetected, but it should be remembered that the disease may be passed on to the next generation.

N.B. Susceptible individuals should ideally be screened for this disease during childhood. Genetic counselling should be offered to all parents of children with the disease, and to adolescents and young adults with the minor form of the disease before becoming parents.

HAEMORRHAGIC ANAEMIAS

Anaemia can result from the loss of red blood cells from the circulating blood through haemorrhage. The condition may result from a large sudden haemorrhage or from prolonged chronic bleeding from one or numerous small sites.

Purpura

Purpura may be the sign of an underlying disease rather than a disease in itself. Characteristic, spontaneous haemorrhages appear in the skin and mucous membrane of the body, causing bruising, petechiae and frank bleeding of the gums, kidneys, intestinal tract, conjunctivae and the brain. The causes of purpura in childhood may be classified under the following headings.

1. Purpura due to primary or secondary platelet deficiency.

2. Purpura due to vascular defects. This may be congenital or acquired.

3. Purpura due to congenital defects of blood plasma, such as prothrombin.

4. Raised capillary pressure.

Purpura due to platelet deficiency

Idiopathic thrombocytopenic purpura. Idiopathic thrombocytopenic purpura occurs without a known cause. Repeated blood transfusions and in some instances platelet transfusions will be given in an attempt to treat the anaemia and control the bleeding which may be most severe and difficult to control. Steroid therapy and prophylactic antibiotics may be given. Some of the more chronic cases may respond well to splenectomy.

Symptomatic thrombocytopenic purpura. Symptomatic thrombocytopenic purpura occurs in such illnesses as leukaemia, aplastic anaemia, rubella syndrome, severe infections and some malignant diseases.

Familial thrombocytopenic purpura. One of the causes of haemorrhage in the newborn is familial thrombocytopenic purpura. Apart from giving platelet transfusions from time to time there is no curative treatment. Splenectomy may be performed when the child is older and this gives good results (see also Haemolytic Disease of the Newborn).

Purpura due to vascular defects

May be either primary or secondary. In primary cases it is thought that a hypersensitivity response may be present which causes temporary permeability of the capillary walls. Henoch-Schönlein's purpura is the most common of this type.

Among secondary types the causes include scurvy, meningococcal meningitis and intolerance to drugs.

Purpura due to lack of essential constituents in the blood plasma

This occurs in haemorrhagic disease of the newborn and obstructive types of jaundice.

Disturbance of clotting mechanism
Haemophilia

Haemophilia is a bleeding disease which occurs almost exclusively in males; the sex-linked genes are transmitted by unaffected females who are carriers. The clotting time is prolonged by a deficiency of factor VIII, the anti-haemophilic globulin.

Freeze-dried human factor VIII or factor IX is available and when patients and their families have adjusted and accepted the treatment for haemophilia the appropriate freeze-dried factors can be self-administered by parents, within the home. The dose is adjusted according to the size of haemorrhage, and hospital management of haemophilia is undertaken in haemophilia centres with the support and advice of the community nursing service.

The haemophiliac child should carry suitable identification at all times to alert first-aiders, medical and nursing staff should accidental trauma occur away from home.

The family health visitor and the school nurse should be kept fully informed of all changes in treatment and care. Genetic counselling should be offered to the parents when the disease is first diagnosed.

Christmas disease

Christmas disease is very similar to haemophilia. The condition is inherited in the same way but is not confined to male sufferers. Heterozygous females may rarely be affected in the same way as males.

The treatment and management is similar to haemophilia.

LEUKAEMIA

Leukaemia is a disease affecting the white blood cells. It is characterized by the presence in the circulating blood of immature leucocytes. The cause is unknown. There are several types of leukaemia depending on the type of cell affected; by far the most common in childhood is acute leukaemia. The disease may occur at any age but is most common between 2 and 5 years.

Acute leukaemia

Acute leukaemia is the most common malignant disease in childhood. It is classified according to the cell type involved.

Acute lymphocytic leukaemia (ALL)—85% of diagnosed cases.

Acute myeloblastic leukaemia (AML)—15% of diagnosed cases.

Nursing management

Nursing action	Explanation
Careful handling to prevent bruising.	Low platelet count creates a tendency to bleed and bruise easily.
Epistaxis relieved with ice packs.	Will reduce blood loss and relieve anxiety.
Blood transfusion should be monitored.	Frequent blood transfusions may result in generalized reactions.
Care taken to reduce the discomfort during the numerous investigations, especially venepunctures and bone marrow punctures.	The disease is diagnosed and monitored by these painful procedures.
Warmth of understanding and recognition of parents' anxieties.	Difficult time for parents adjusting to their child's illness.
Involving the support of the health visitor and social worker.	Within the home the child and family will require help and support.
Encourage the normal family lifestyle despite the long-term nature of the illness—education, play activities, hobbies, etc.	The continuity of 'normality' will give reassurance to the child and his family.

Drug therapy

Without the use of modern drugs children with acute leukaemia would die within a few months. By using steroids, cytotoxic drugs and antimetabolite drugs, remission of the disease may be obtained for a variable period of time. The effect may be dramatic, with the child starting to eat well and taking part in all his former activities. It should be remembered that these drugs are also toxic to healthy cells and are used with great care. The white cell count may fall considerably and therefore secondary infection may

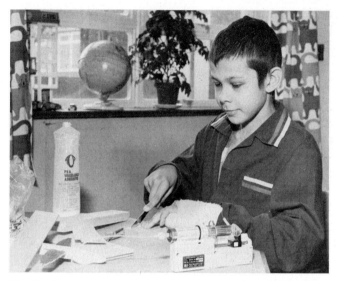

Fig. 30. Cytotoxic drugs administered by clockwork pump allows for normal activities to continue.

occur. For this reason prophylactic antibiotics may be prescribed. The child, as far as possible, being protected from infection.

Intrathecal methotrexate together with radiotherapy to the meninges to prevent leukaemic secondaries being deposited around the brain are part of the routine management of acute leukaemia. Alopecia is an unavoidable side-effect of cytotoxic drug therapy and radiotherapy. A wig may be provided. Long-term care may necessitate a further course of drug therapy. The average survival of these children is from 2½ years to 5 years and many of the five year survivors may be cured.

Usually admission to hospital takes place to confirm the diagnosis and establish treatment and remission. Thereafter admission is kept to a minimum, the continuing care and treatment being carried out as an outpatient with close liaison with the primary health care team and, in particular, the health visitor.

HODGKIN'S DISEASE

Hodgkin's disease affects the lymphoid tissues of the body, causing enlargement of lymph glands. Any group (or groups) of glands may be affected but it is usually the cervical or axillary glands that are involved. The disease is rare, and is most unusual under the age of 5 years.

The child is listless, anaemic and progressively becomes more ill. Waves of recurrent low grade pyrexia or 'Pel-Ebstein' fever is usually present. Remissions may occur. There is no cure for this disease but life can be prolonged by therapy. Treatment includes deep X-ray therapy and the administration of cell-destroying drugs, e.g. cyclophosphamide and chlorambucil.

Further reading

FLEMING, A. F. (1982) *Sickle-Cell Disease*. London: Churchill Livingstone.

JONES, P. (1974) *Living with Haemophilia*. Lancaster: Medical & Technical Publishers.

JONES, P. (1977) *Haemophilia Home Therapy*. London: Churchill Livingstone.

MILLER, D. R. (1978) *Smith's Blood Diseases in Infancy*, 4th edn. St. Louis: C. V. Mosby.

WILLOUGHBY, M. L. N. (1977) *Paediatric Haematology*. London: Churchill Livingstone.

9 Disorders of the alimentary system

Daily oral toilet is as important in young children as in the older ones and in adults. The popular belief that the first teeth are unimportant as they will soon be replaced by the permanent ones, is erroneous, and the nurse should make it her duty to teach the child—and through him the mother—good habits with regard to dental care.

Cleaning the teeth with an attractive toothbrush and nice-tasting toothpaste can be a pleasant part of the morning and evening toilet. Very young children are often reluctant to open their mouth, and so make effective cleaning impossible. It is therefore often best to let the child chew a piece of raw apple at least once a day as soon as the first teeth have come through—a most effective way of keeping the teeth healthy and clean.

THE MOUTH

Observations on the condition of a patient's mouth will often assist in diagnosis and treatment. Of special importance are the following points:

1. *Dry lips and tongue* which will be present in mouth-breathers and in those with high fevers and dehydration. At the same time the tongue will often be thickly coated.

2. *Herpes* which is often seen in patients with colds, high fevers and pneumonia. These small vesicles, grouped on a patch of inflammation around the mouth, are sometimes also called fever blisters.

3. *Pallor of the lips* which is caused by anaemia and may be a sign of loss of blood.

Important odours which a nurse should recognize include:

A sweet smell, where acetone is present.

The smell of stale blood in cases of bleeding from the tonsil bed or from the stomach.

Offensive smells which may be due to the presence of pus, as in retropharyngeal abscess and bronchiectasis.

A faecal odour in intestinal obstruction.

A urinary smell in uraemia.

A foul smell from the mouth occurs in the late stages of leukaemia.

Specific smells when poisons have been swallowed.

Treatment of any of these symptoms depends on their cause, but in all cases of sickness careful mouth toilet is an essential of good nursing.

Herpes simplex

Herpes simplex is a virus infection which causes eruptions of vesicles. A common site is the lips in febrile illnesses causing swelling and blisters. The latter dry off and leave thick, uncomfortable crusts. The lesions are best treated by drying them up with dusting powder or applying Neocortef ointment. Dabbing the blisters with methylated spirit is painful and for that reason particularly unsuitable for children.

Catarrhal, aphthous and ulcerative stomatitis

Catarrhal, aphthous and ulcerative stomatitis are varying degrees of generalized inflammation of the mouth. There is swelling and inflammation of the gums, coupled with ulcers on the mucous lining of the mouth. The tongue is coated and there is a foul smell. The patient seems ill, the temperature is often raised, he refuses his food and shows intense misery. Frequently these children are debilitated and come from poor homes.

A swab is taken to determine the causative organism. In

many cases of aphthous stomatitis, the cause is the ultra-microscopic virus of herpes simplex.

Nursing management

As these children dribble saliva because swallowing is so painful, the chin should be protected by applying Vaseline. A dish or a piece of absorbent material can often be arranged to catch the saliva. The application of Vaseline will give some relief from this painful condition by protecting the ulcer from rubbing on the gums or teeth. Benzocaine lozenges to suck will also help. For persistent ulcers, a light touch with a silver nitrate stick or Bonjela ointment may shorten the course of the ulcer. For Vincent's angina oral penicillin is usually effective, alternatively oral metronidazole (Flagyl) may be given. Very young children may have to have their arms restrained to prevent them from putting their fingers in their mouths. It is usual to carry out barrier nursing.

Bland, cool fluids containing plenty of glucose should be given at first and later the diet should contain extra milk and nourishment. Vitamins are important, but concentrated orange juice should be avoided as it stings on the open lesions. Groats are often enjoyed and can be fortified by addition of an egg. Teeth and tonsils should be inspected and, if necessary, treatment or tonsillectomy carried out to eliminate septic foci.

There is a danger of aspiration pneumonia from inhaled saliva. Drainage of saliva may require to be encouraged by raising the foot of the bed.

Gingivitis

Swollen, bleeding gums, may be present in general oral infections. They occur in ulcerative stomatitis, scurvy and in leukaemia, but sometimes may merely be due to poor oral hygiene. Careful mouth toilet and a well-balanced diet are essential. Certain drugs taken over a long period may also cause gingivitis.

Teething

Gentle mouth toilet should be carried out. A mild analgesic, such as Disprin or a Junior Aspirin may be ordered for relief of pain and there is no point in withholding this simple analgesic. A little comforting and nursing will help to soothe these children. Teething rings, which the infant can bite on, relieve the discomfort and there is nothing against them, provided they are kept clean and safely tied to the cot to prevent them from falling onto the floor.

Thrush

Thrush is caused by the fungus *Candida (Monilia) albicans*. It is mostly seen in bottle-fed babies and is a highly contagious condition. White or grey patches appear on the inside of the cheeks and lips, on the roof of the mouth and on the tongue and cannot be removed without damaging the mucous membrane. The baby will be reluctant to take his feed.

Thrush can be prevented by scrupulous cleanliness, especially with regard to feeding utensils, and by keeping the mucous membrane moist in case of high fever or dehydration. Babies on broad spectrum antibiotics are particularly prone to thrush because the drug kills the organisms which are normally present in the mouth and which can control the antibiotic resistant *Candida albicans*. Vitamin B should always be given with these antibiotics.

Nursing management

Because the condition is highly contagious, strict barrier nursing is essential. Feed bottles must not be returned to the common feed kitchen until sterilized.

The infection is treated by giving an oral antibiotic called Nystatin. The dose is 1 ml (100 000 units) four times a day after feeding until all signs of thrush disappear. The solution is usually dropped directly onto the tongue. Nystatin should not be used for more than 7 days after dispensing. If prolonged treatment is required a newly prepared solution should be ordered. Alternative methods of treatment are: painting the mouth with a 0.5% aqueous solution of gentian violet, or a 1 : 10 000 solution of thiomersal (Merthiolate). The treatment being carried out three times a day.

Complications

Infection may spread throughout the gastro-intestinal tract and cause thrush septicaemia, a very serious condition. Severe cases are treated by giving hydroxystilbamidine in a solution of glucose and saline by intravenous infusion. Buttock lesions should be treated with a local application of gentian violet, 0.5%, and the baby nursed with exposed buttocks.

Nurses can assist in the prevention of thrush by teaching mothers adequate, easy methods of hygiene in infant feeding.

Tongue tie

Occasionally a child cannot stretch his tongue sufficiently to make it protrude beyond the teeth. This may cause feeding and speech difficulty so that the fraenum has to be cut in a minor operation. Mild degrees of tongue tie usually right themselves as the child grows older.

THE OESOPHAGUS AND STOMACH

Vomiting

Vomiting in the neonatal period should never be treated lightly. If it is persistent, recurrent, forceful or copious, admission to hospital should be arranged at once. Immediate operation for an obstruction may be necessary, and expert observations may prove life saving. In childhood the causes of vomiting are very varied (see Table 4) and

Table 4. The causes of vomiting in childhood

Causes	Age	Content of the vomit	Remarks
Underfeeding	0–3 months	Recently taken feed	The hungry infant cries, swallows air and gulps the feed when offered
Indiscretion in diet	All ages	Undigested food	Milky curd in infancy
Congenital abnormalities	Infancy	Milk, mucus	Effortless or projectile
Pyloric stenosis	2 weeks to 4 months	Curd, mucus, occasionally blood	Projectile
Gastritis	All ages	Food, mucus, blood	Colicky pain often presents
At the onset of fevers	Young children	No characteristic	Accompanied by rise in temperature
Acute appendicitis	All ages	Food at first, bile later	Associated with abdominal pain
Toxic illness	All ages	Food, gastric fluid	Quickly causes dehydration
Whooping cough	All ages	Food and mucus	During or just after meals. After attack of coughing
Diabetes mellitus	All ages	Food	Heralds impending coma
Renal diseases	All ages	Fluid gastric contents	Mostly in late stages of the illness
Poisoning	All ages	Gastric contents	Must be saved with special care
Intolerance to drugs	All ages	Gastric contents	e.g. Salicylates. The drugs may have to be discontinued

Nervous conditions	All ages	Watery	Excitement, anxiety, habit
Cyclical vomiting	After age of 2 years	Food at first, later gastric fluid only	Severe, general disturbance. Ketosis, may last several days
Mechanical	All ages	Gastric contents	May result from finger sucking, enlarged tonsils, mucopus in nasopharynx, air swallowing
Oesophageal reflux	Infancy	Feed, mucus, sometimes blood	e.g. Hiatus hernia
Intracranial pressure	All ages	Not related to taking food	Gastric contents, projectile, without warning
If associated with meningitis, constipation is often an accompanying feature

some children seem to vomit at the slightest provocation and show little or no concern about it. Nonetheless, the nurse should remember that vomiting in most cases entails considerable effort and the child may feel dizzy, faint, cold and miserable. The nurse should always remain with the child, protecting the bedclothes and placing the patient in a comfortable position, and if necessary drawing the curtains around the bed. The patient may find it comforting if the nurse holds her hand on his forehead and supports any recent abdominal wound. When the attack is over, the patient should be given a mouthwash, or have his teeth cleaned, and be left comfortable. Persistent vomiting may cause considerable loss of fluid and replacement by a parenteral route is sometimes necessary.

The vomit should always be inspected before it is discarded and an entry should be made on the patient's chart. The amount should be measured, the reaction tested with litmus paper, and the time and relation to mealtimes recorded. The nurse should notice whether the vomit is effortless, or forcible and projectile in nature. The presence of curds, blood, excess mucus, bile or foreign bodies should be reported at once.

Gastritis

The causes of acute irritation or inflammation of the gastric mucosa range from unsuitable diet; swallowing infected material; e.g. pus from sinusitis, or dental caries causing incomplete mastication; intolerance of drugs ; swallowing an irritant such as a poison; gastroenteritis or chronic dilatation, as in pyloric stenosis.

Nursing management

As gastritis is, as a rule, a symptom of some other

disturbance, the underlying cause must be found and appropriately treated.

If old enough, the child may complain of discomfort, nausea and vomiting. The vomit may contain mucus, or specks of fresh blood. Vomiting frequently relieves the distension and discomfort. Ordinary food is omitted from the diet for a few days to reduce irritation to the gastric mucosa. Clear fluids, mildly flavoured, are encouraged to prevent and correct any dehydration. The child generally has a poor appetite. The return to a full diet should be gradual. Lightly boiled eggs, soups, toast and ice-cream are suitable as soon as the child is ready for more solid food.

When the illness is severe or long-standing, gastric lavage may be beneficial. Oral hygiene should be given frequently to the dry mouth and furred tongue.

Congenital hypertrophic pyloric stenosis

Congenital hypertrophic pyloric stenosis is due to the thickening of the pyloric sphincter, causing a narrowing of the lumen. Signs of obstruction, gastritis and malnutrition develop.

Pyloric stenosis develops soon after birth and symptoms are first noticed at the age of 2–6 weeks. Mild cases or those which show late symptoms may improve spontaneously at the age of about 4 months, but early and severe cases require medical or surgical treatment.

Diagnosis

Diagnosis is often delayed as varying feeds are tried in an attempt to stop the baby from vomiting. At each change a temporary improvement may take place but vomiting and loss of weight soon recur and eventually the presence of pyloric stenosis is suspected.

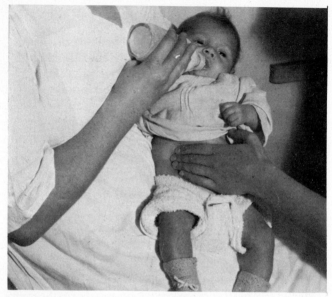

Fig. 31. Pyloric stenosis. The doctor is feeling the swelling and watching for visible peristalsis. Note the relaxed position and the way in which the abdomen has been exposed by the nurse, although the rest of the baby is being kept warm.

Pre-operative nursing management

Nursing action	Explanation
Observation of vomiting. The amount, content and frequency should be recorded.	Large projectile vomits containing curds from previous feeds and flecks of blood from gastritis.
Intake and output fluid balance-chart maintained.	The vomiting causes dehydration and the urine is dark and scanty. The skin is dry and fontanelle is sunken.
Assist doctor by administering a feed whilst the abdomen is examined for pyloric nodule.	Peristaltic action during feeding causes the pyloric muscle to contract.

Nursing action	Explanation
Care of the intravenous infusion, and blood specimen taken for analysis of blood chemistry.	Replacement of fluids to correct dehydration and blood chemistry. The loss of chlorides in the vomit has a serious effect in altering the blood chemistry. Plasma bicarbonates are high and there is an increase in the non-protein nitrogen in the blood and urine. The toxic state (alkalosis) requires rectifying without delay and before operation.
Gastric lavage once or twice daily.	Clears the stomach of stale milk, curds and mucus. The tube is left in situ immediately before operation.
Normal preparation for theatre.	Surgery under general anaesthetic is the usual method of treatment.

Post-operative nursing management

Details of feeding vary from one hospital to another but the fundamental principles remain the same. If the baby is breast-fed every effort should be made to help the mother keep the supply going. The first feed offered to the baby may be 5 ml of boiled water. The baby may then, 4 hours post-operatively, be offered the breast for 1–2 min. The baby will then be given a breast feed 3-hourly, gradually increasing the time allowed for feeding, and thus increasing the amount of feed taken.

Alternatively the baby may follow a typical post-operative pyloric regime as follows:

Hours post-operation

4–8	5 ml dextrose hourly
8–10	10 ml dextrose hourly
10–12	10 ml half-strength milk feeds hourly
12–18	15 ml half-strength milk feeds 2-hourly
18–24	30 ml half-strength milk feeds 2-hourly

24–30	30 ml full-strength milk feeds 2-hourly
30–36	45 ml full-strength milk feeds 2-hourly
36–42	60 ml full-strength milk feeds 3-hourly
42–48	75 ml full-strength milk feeds 3-hourly

After 48 hours, the baby may be expected to take normal feeds according to expected weight. One or two vomits during the early post-operative period are not uncommon, and there may be a little delay in establishing normal gastric peristalsis. The problem is usually resolved or relieved with a further gastric washout; the baby is usually well and gaining weight by 72 hours, and may be discharged home once he is taking full feeds for 24 hours.

Gastric lavage

The equipment required for gastric lavage in young children differs from that used for adults only in some minor detail. As the nasogastric tube can be connected directly to the funnel, neither extra length of tubing, nor a size 8–10 French gauge connection are needed. This eliminates extra weight to manipulate. To stop the flow the tube is often doubled back on itself instead of using a gate clip, and the rate of flow is regulated by raising or lowering the tube and funnel. Instead of the open type funnel a cylindrical upright glass funnel is used and any gastric contents or lavage fluid should be allowed to run back into the funnel and not emptied directly into a receiver or bucket. In that way a comparison can be made between the amounts run in and returned. This is important on account of the small amounts involved and the danger of causing distension and colic if too much fluid is allowed to run into the stomach or to accumulate there.

Babies and young children should be securely wrapped in a blanket to avoid any struggle, as little cooperation can be expected. The tube should be measured from the bridge of the nose to the lower end of the sternum to give an idea how far the tube needs to be passed in order to enter the stomach. The point is reached when the mark made on the tube, after measuring, reaches the level of the dental arch.

Children cannot be expected to assist with the passing of the tube by swallowing or deep breathing and it is best to feed the tube gently, but firmly along the floor of the mouth after lubricating it with a little sterile water. The assisting nurse, or a parent if present, may steady the child's head or support the chin as this helps to reduce the tickling sensation and excessive retching. After seeing gastric residue rise in the funnel, or after testing some resting juice which has been obtained by siphon action for reaction on litmus paper, fluid [e.g. normal saline at a temperature of 37.2°–37.8°C (99°–100°F)] is run into the stomach. The amount will vary according to the age and size of the patient but in the majority of cases it is satisfactory to allow one funnel-full to run in at a time and then to siphon the fluid back. Gastric lavage in children should always be supervised by a trained nurse who will be able to give advice from her own experience as to the correct quantity of fluid which should be used. By raising or lowering the funnel, fluid can be siphoned back. At the end of the procedure the nurse should make sure that no fluid is left in the stomach.

Nasogastric tube feed

When giving a feed by nasogastric tube, the technique and equipment are essentially the same as for a gastric lavage. The size of tube used is usually a smaller bore.

At the end of the feed the funnel should be allowed to empty down to the juncture of the funnel and tube, before adding a small amount of water. This reduces the mixing of fluid and feed to a minimum and also ensures that the baby gets all the feed. If the tube is withdrawn before it has emptied completely, as much as 14 g of feed may be lost, a

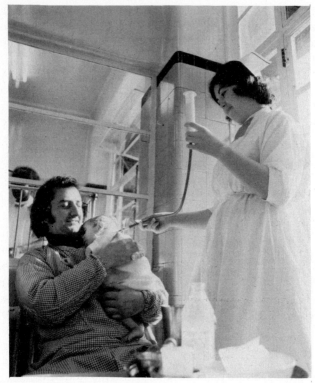

Fig. 32. Proud father holding infant son during naso-oesophageal feed.

considerable proportion of the total if the small amounts sometimes involved in infant feeding are considered. Furthermore, as long as there is any fluid in the tube, there is always a danger that some may be aspirated into the trachea as the tube passes the larynx on withdrawal. As an additional safety measure, and in order to prevent this from happening, it is considered wise to pinch the tube whilst withdrawing it. The tube should always be withdrawn fairly quickly, and in one steady pull.

On completion of the feed, sometimes the tube is left in situ unspigotted to allow free drainage and prevent distension of the stomach.

Hiatus hernia

Hiatus hernia is a special type of diaphragmatic hernia. The abnormality is caused by a defect in the muscles forming the diaphragm so that these do not fit closely around the distal end of the oesophagus, and part of the stomach is pulled through the opening into the thoracic cavity. Sphincter control is impaired and there is a constant reflux of gastric secretions and food into the oesophagus.

Nursing management

As time goes on the baby vomits mucus, food and even blood soon after feeds, and later at any time. He fails to gain weight as much food is lost in this way, and if the condition is not corrected, ulceration of the lining of the oesophagus results. The milky vomit may become streaked with blood. Treatment consists of keeping the baby constantly in an upright position and this position should be maintained day and night, even when the baby is bathed or nursed. In this way the stomach is kept below the diaphragm and vomiting made more difficult by force of gravity. It may help to thicken feeds with Nestargel or with Bengor's.

Feeds should be given slowly; this allows the oesophagitis to resolve by preventing regurgitation and causing some gain in weight. The diagnosis is confirmed by barium swallow and radiographs. In most instances the hernia is repaired by surgery.

The stomach is returned to the abdominal cavity and the defect in the diaphragm repaired. The surgical approach is usually through the abdomen but may be through the chest.

As soon as condition permits, the child is nursed in a sitting position, particularly after feeds.

Abnormalities of the oesophagus

There are a number of variants of the abnormalities of the oesophagus, and these may or may not involve the trachea.

1. Tracheo-oesophageal fistula without associated atresia of the oesophagus.
2. Oesophageal atresia, i.e. the oesophagus is not continuous but neither end communicates with the trachea.
3. Oesophageal atresia with associated tracheo-oesophageal fistula.

These abnormalities occur most commonly in low birth-weight babies. There is often a history of hydramnios during pregnancy. Symptoms vary according to the abnormality.

1. In the case of tracheo-oesophageal fistula not associated with atresia of the oesophagus, gastric reflux will cause inhalation of secretions and of hydrochloric acid from the stomach into the trachea causing ulceration of the mucous lining.
2. As neither saliva nor oral fluids can pass into the stomach the blind pouch of the proximal end of the oesophagus soon fills up and spills over, causing coughing and choking as fluid enters the lungs. Inhalation pneumonia results.
3. When atresia associated with a communication between oesophagus and trachea is present, there is again obvious danger of reflux and inhalation of secretions and any feed that might be given.

Pre-operative management

Nursing action	Explanation
Gentle aspiration of the naso-pharynx and mouth at regular intervals and when required.	Because the infant is unable to swallow secretions, coughing and choking occur.
Continuous or intermittent suction to a tube residing in the blind oesophageal pouch.	It is unwise to lower the head end of the cot as this would encourage reflux of stomach secretions into the lungs.
No oral feeds.	
Care of the intravenous infusion.	To maintain hydration.
Normal preparation for operation.	

Post-operative management

When the oesophageal blind ends are in close proximity to each other, a simple anastomosis may be carried out through a thoracotomy. This one-stage repair leaves a transanastomotic tube in situ for a week and tube feeding commences after 24 hours. The first oral feed will be a few drops of sterile water, given after seven days, the patency of the anastomosis being tested.

Post-operatively, the baby should be handled as little as possible and it is convenient to use an incubator. If the proximal and distal ends of the oesophagus are too far apart to be brought together, a graft to bridge the gap is necessary. The graft may consist of some inert material or may be taken from the patient's own intestinal tract. It is usually necessary to do the repair in two stages. In that event the proximal end of the oesophagus is brought to the surface at the base of the neck, and through it secretions are discharged. A 'sham feed' of clear fluid is given at the same time as gastrostomy feed, so that the infant associates sucking and swallowing with the pleasure of a full stomach. This makes it easier to establish normal feeding when reconstruction of the oesophagus is completed. A gastrostomy is established through which the child can be fed.

Feeds given through a gastrostomy tube are given slowly to avoid distension. The funnel is not raised above the height of the baby so that the feed flows gently and gas can escape when necessary. Special care is given to the skin surrounding the gastrostomy opening, and to the mouth.

Hydration and electrolyte balance are maintained by an intravenous infusion before and after surgery. Gentle physiotherapy is carried out to prevent chest complications.

THE INTESTINE

Constipation

Infrequent bowel actions are unlikely to be harmful, provided the stools are soft and passed without causing pain or distress. Few paediatricians are in favour of giving enemas or aperients and regular dosing should be discouraged unless specifically prescribed by the doctor.

Constipation is a symptom rather than a disease in itself; the underlying cause should be found and treatment given accordingly. True constipation can, however, be responsible for a number of symptoms such as furred tongue, anorexia and vomiting, poor general circulation and sluggishness, restless sleep and bedwetting.

True constipation, that is to say dry, hard faeces passed with difficulty, may be due to a long list of causes including those mentioned below:

In young babies: underfeeding due to inadequate fluid or calorie intake or a failure of lactation.

Congenital abnormalities: these may hold up the food or faeces or inhibit peristalsis. Among such conditions are congenital pyloric stenosis, intestinal atresia, stricture of the anus, Hirschsprung's disease, hypothyroidism, mental deficiency and atonia due to muscular dystrophy or debility.

Painful defecation: this may be due to local causes, e.g. anal fissure, which makes the child hold back the stool to avoid pain.

Parenteral causes: illnesses which result in a reduction in the circulating fluid volume such as febrile illness and conditions which cause oedema.

Psychological factors: these, or faulty habit training, may lead to infrequent bowel actions and so cause hard stools and painful defecation. Such psychological factors include maternal anxiety.

Nursing management

Dietary adjustments may be all that is necessary. For infants a small amount of sugar added to a feed, or drinks of boiled water in between ordinary feeds, as well as extra orange juice, may prove sufficient. In older children a diet rich in roughage and adequate exercise; regular habit training should be encouraged. The child old enough to cooperate should have an unhurried time on the toilet planned into his morning routine. Allbran, wholemeal bread, fresh fruit, green vegetables and prune juice are palatable and suitable high roughage additions to the daily diet.

Occasionally it is found that constipation has developed because the lavatory in the child's home is situated in a cold, dark or isolated part of a tenement building or house, so that the child is frightened of going there on his own. Alternatively, the toilet seat may be too high and, as the child's feet cannot touch the ground, he is frightened of falling in. Lack of time before leaving for school may be another, easily remedied cause of chronic constipation. Lack of exercise leading to poor circulation and muscle tone should be corrected. Television viewing has contributed to physical inactivity in recent years and all types of sport should be encouraged as a healthy counterbalance.

Severe cases of long-standing may need initial treatment by colonic lavage or enemas.

Anal fissure

The severe pain experienced on defaecation should be minimized by keeping the faeces soft with the aid of a correct diet and mild laxatives. Local anaesthetizing ointment such as amethocaine may be used.

Constipation with overflow

This is a term used for leakage of decomposed faeces around a mass of impacted faecal matter. The condition is mainly seen in children with psychiatric disturbances or children who are mentally handicapped. Treatment includes patient toilet training, aperients and, occasionally manual removal under anaesthetic. For treatment to be successful it is important to find out the underlying cause. In the meantime the patient's mother, exasperated by the constant soiling of clothes will need support and sympathy in order to gain her cooperation in treating the condition.

Observation of faeces

Although the observation of faeces is an important duty of every nurse, it is of immeasurable value in paediatric nursing. Children are often unable to describe symptoms accurately, and the abnormal stool preserved for inspection by an experienced ward sister or medical officer may frequently lead to the establishment of a previously doubtful diagnosis. The nurse should note such points as the colour, consistency, odour, shape and frequency of the stools. Any abnormal constituents such as blood, mucus or foreign bodies should be noted and any complaints of pain on passing the stool, treated as being significant (see Table 5).

Table 5. Types of stools in infancy and childhood

Description	Usual occurrence	Colour	Odour	Consistency	Frequency	Composition	Reaction
Meconium	First 2–3 days after birth	Tarry, changing to greenish-black	None	Semi-solid	3–6 daily	Normal	Neutral
Changing stools	Approx. 3rd–6th day of life	Dark green changing to yellow	None	Soft	5–8 daily	Normal	Acid
Breast-milk stools	In breast-fed babies	Mustard colour	Characteristic	Soft homogeneous	5–6 daily	Normal	Acid
Cow's-milk stools	In artificially fed babies	A pale yellow-grey	Musty	Semi-formed, bulky	4–5 daily	Normal	Alkaline
Mixed feeding	In toddlers	Brown	Slight	Formed	1–2 daily	Normal	Varies
High protein content	In infancy	Grey	Sour and offensive	Dry and crumbling	1–2 daily	Excess protein	Alkaline
High fat content	e.g. Coeliac disease	Grey, clay coloured	Offensive	Bulky, greasy	Several daily	Excess fat deficient in bile	Acid
High carbohydrate content	In infancy	Green	Slightly offensive	Relaxed, frothy	Frequent	Fermented faeces	Very acid

Table 5. Types of stools in infancy and childhood—cont.

Description	Usual occurrence	Colour	Odour	Consistency	Frequency	Composition	Reaction
Soapy stools	Digestive disturbances	White	Offensive	Pasty	Several daily	Excess fat or deficient in bile	Neutral
Melaena	Swallowed blood, intestinal bleeding	Tarry-black	Characteristic sweet	Soft	Varies	Blood	Alkaline
Intestinal hurry	Gastrointestinal infections	Bright green	Characteristic offensive	Fluid, relaxed	Many times daily	Unconverted bile	Neutral
	Disaccharide intolerance	Green-brown		Fluid	Many times	Reducing substances	Acid
Hunger stools	Infancy	Dark green	None or sour	Small, dry	Frequent	Large proportion of mucus-bile	Acid
Over-feeding	Infancy	Bright green	Offensive	Frothy, fermenting	Frequent	Excess fat and carbohydrate	Very acid

Intestinal infections	Gastro-enteritis	Pale green	Characteristic offensive	Soft or liquid	Very frequent	Partially digested food, mucus	Varies
Fresh blood	1 Anal fissure 2 Ulcerative colitis 3 Dysentery 4 Rectal polyp	Bright red	1 None 2} 3} Offensive 4 None	1 Hard 2} 3} Liquid 4 Normal	1 Infrequent 2} 3} Frequent 4 Normal	1 Normal 2} Mucus 3} bile, blood 4 Normal and streaks of blood	Alkaline
Red currant jelly stool	Intussus-ception	Bright red	None	Jelly-like	1 or 2 isolated stools	Mucus, blood	Neutral
Pea-soup stool	Typhoid	Green	Offensive	Liquid	Very frequent	Mucus, pus, blood	—
Pus, mucus	Pelvic abscess	Normal or green, streaked with pus	Offensive	Relaxed	Once after rupture of abscess into bowel	Pus, mucus	—

Collection of specimens

The collection of faecal matter for investigation does not differ from that in adult nursing but, in the case of 24-hour specimens for very young children, a specially constructed chair may have to be used or the napkin lined with thin plastic.

The handling of bedpans and pots should at all times be reduced to a minimum. Soiled napkins should be saved with the corners tucked underneath the part on which the stool lies when first taken off the baby, placed in a receiver and covered with a glass plate. It is now ready for easy inspection. Any doubtful stool should always be saved and kept available during the paediatrician's round.

Intestinal obstruction

Intestinal obstruction in childhood may be due to congenital abnormalities, strangulated hernia, intussusception, volvulus, a swallowed foreign body or pressure from a tumour. The classical symptoms are the same as in adults, namely vomiting, pain, absolute constipation and abdominal distension (Fig. 33). Urgent operation to relieve the obstruction is necessary otherwise there is a danger that the constriction of the blood supply may lead to gangrene of the strangulated portion of the gut, and the continued vomiting

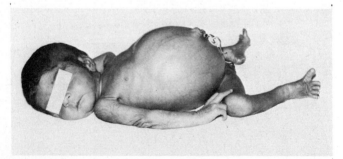

Fig. 33. Young infant with gross abdominal distension due to intestinal obstruction.

may result in dehydration and loss of electrolytes. A nasogastric tube is passed and the stomach contents aspirated before giving an anaesthetic. An intravenous infusion will be necessary.

Duodenal atresia

Duodenal obstruction in the neonate is due to narrowing or absence of the duodenum lumen. There is often a history of hydramnios in pregnancy and other abnormalities may be present.

Vomiting starts within 4 hours of birth and the vomit may contain bile.

Nursing management

The infant pre- and post-operatively requires the usual care after major surgery for intestinal obstruction. To avoid strain on the anastomosis, the transanastomotic tube may be in situ via the nasogastric route or alternatively through a gastrostomy. Feeding, either orally or through the trans-anastomotic tube, is commenced when bowel sounds are heard. Feeds given into the jejunum are given in very small amounts, at approximately 1 ml/min.

Volvulus

A different kind of obstruction occurs in volvulus, when a loop of bowel gets twisted round itself causing complete obstruction, but symptoms and treatment are similar to the ones described above. After opening the abdomen, the site of volvulus is sought and the gut untwisted and anchored to the peritoneum. Resection and anastomosis are rarely necessary.

Intussusception

Intussusception, a partial or total obstruction of the bowel, is caused by invagination of a piece of bowel into the bowel beyond it.

Intussusception is one of the most urgent emergencies of early childhood, though on occasions repeated attacks occur, which rectify themselves. Acute intussusception is seen usually at the time the infant starts a weaning diet and it is possible that irritation of the bowel causes a small area of inflammation and oedema is the ileocaecal or ileocolic region, which is the starting point of the telescoping of the bowel. A high proportion of children show signs of a recent virus infection causing oedema of the lymphoid tissue of the bowel. This swelling is then the starting point of the telescoping. A portion of the bowel becomes invaginated and is dragged onwards towards the rectum by peristaltic movement. If the diagnosis is doubtful, a barium enema may be ordered to confirm the diagnosis and on occasions this has the effect of reducing the intussusception, so that surgery becomes unnecessary.

Nursing management

The infant is, as a rule, a well-nourished healthy baby of 4 months to 2 years. The mother will explain that he suddenly seemed to have severe abdominal colic which made him draw up his legs and that these pains had been recurring at intervals, between which the baby seemed normal and contented. At first the pain may recur every hour or $1/2$ hr but it soon becomes more frequent and its severity causes shock, with pallor, sweating and a cold clammy skin. The baby soon becomes exhausted. At first a normal stool may be passed but this is followed by complete constipation due to the obstruction, except for the passage of blood-stained mucus—the typical 'red currant jelly stool'. Vomiting may occur but is not a constant symptom.

Nothing is offered orally because the infant may require surgery. A barium enema may be performed to assist diagnosis and may result in reducing the intussusception, preventing surgical intervention. More usually an operation is performed and the infant is prepared for theatre, passing a nasogastric tube to aspirate the stomach contents to avoid inhalation of vomited food. The abdominal skin, the umbilicus and the groins are washed with soap and water, or the child is bathed if the condition permits.

Post-operative care is usually straightforward. Fluids are given in small amounts—some hospitals start on a 'pyloric schedule'—but in most cases the child can return to a light, normal diet within 3 or 4 days. Any vomiting, the passage of flatus and the first stool are reported as they are an important guide to treatment. The wound is often left exposed, or covered with a small dressing, and the stitches are usually removed on the eighth and tenth day respectively.

Restriction of bowel

Whenever extensive resection of bowel has been carried out, the child's diet will have to be carefully regulated as abnormalities of digestion and absorption result. Disturbances of growth, electrolyte balance, blood formation and vitamin absorption must all be prevented.

Acute appendicitis

There are few conditions in childhood that present a more confusing picture than acute appendicitis. Among the conditions which may lead to this diagnosis erroneously are tonsillitis, mesenteric adenitis, urinary tract infections, pneumonia, diaphragmatic pleurisy, meningitis, anaphylactoid purpura, dysentery, gastroenteritis, and premenstrual pain. Assessment of all symptoms and sometimes a period of careful observation will, however, establish the correct diagnosis. Because of the extensive examination necessary to establish the correct diagnosis, the nurse may have to be prepared for an ear, nose and throat and a neurological examination, a rectal swab, a clean specimen of urine, blood picture and chest X-ray.

Acute appendicitis is rare before the age of 2 years and most common at 5–12 years. The onset may be insidious with anorexia, listlessness, nausea or one or two attacks of vomiting and constipation. Alternatively the child may become acutely ill with little warning. The temperature may rise to between 37.2° and 38.4°C (99°–101°F), the pulse may become rapid and the expression, anxious. The tongue is furred and there is halitosis. The child is irritable and resents being touched or examined. If the appendix lies deep in the pelvis—pelvic appendix—the symptoms may include frequency of micturition and diarrhoea due to irritation, and if the appendix is retrocaecal the abdominal signs will be masked and diagnosis made very difficult.

Pain may be vague and intermittent to begin with but it gradually moves to the para-umbilical region and within 12 hours settles in the right iliac fossa.

On examination there is guarding and tenderness, and rectal examination causes the patient to flinch or cry out in pain as the finger points towards the right side. Abdominal rigidity may be caused by cold or general protest and for that reason it is particularly important in children that the doctor's hands should be warm and that a moment or two should be spent in gaining the child's confidence. Occasionally a sedative has to be given before a satisfactory examination can be carried out. If a white cell count is done, it is found to be raised to as much as 30 000 white cells/mm^3 (mainly polymorphonuclear cells).

Once diagnosis has been made, operation should not be delayed. Peritonitis occurs readily as the poorly developed peritoneum is less resistant to infection in a child than in later life, and infection does not localize well in childhood. The appendix wall is thin and the appendix perforates more often than in adults and with more serious results. Operation and after-care are the same for children as for adults and in an uneventful case the child can be expected to be up for bedmaking on the first day after operation and playing happily in the wards on the second day.

Complications: perforated appendix

Acute appendicitis which cannot be diagnosed or treated in time, may lead to perforation and set up peritonitis or form a pelvic abscess. When perforation has occurred, there may, for a time, appear to be some improvement in the child's condition. The pain subsides, he seems more relaxed and may fall asleep. However the temperature and pulse rate will rise and the rigidity will spread and, after a few hours, it becomes evident that he is seriously ill and in spite of operation, complications have now become unavoidable.

Peritonitis

The course of peritonitis is now usually controlled by chemotherapy, but severe cases do occur and merit description, as good nursing care has considerable bearing on a satisfactory outcome. Peritonitis may be caused by surgical emergencies such as a ruptured appendix, perforation of the bowel due to ulcerative colitis, ascending infection from the vagina and infection in the blood stream. In newborn babies the infection may enter via the umbilicus. The causative organisms include the staphylococcus, *Escherichia coli* (bacterium), the tubercle bacillus; gonococcus and pneumococcus.

In the case of a perforated appendix, the causative organism is usually *Escherichia coli* and the fluid in the peritoneal cavity soon becomes infected. The onset is mostly very acute.

Nursing management. The temperature rises to between 39.4° and 40.6°C (103°–105°F), the tongue is furred, the child vomits and complains of abdominal pain or draws up his legs. In very young patients this pain may not be localized as it is in older children. Respirations are rapid and shallow, the diaphragm being immobilized as the movements of the abdomen cause pain, but the arms are thrown out above the head in order to increase the respiratory capacity. The colour of the skin is grey, with a malar flush, and the eyes bright but sunken and surrounded by dark rings. The legs are drawn up in a 'frog position' in an attempt to relieve abdominal pain. Free fluid will be present in the abdominal cavity and the abdomen is rigid. The picture is that of severe toxaemia.

Children suffering from such a serious illness need expert and continuous nursing care. The mouth will have to be treated frequently, the position changed and pillows turned in order to encourage rest and sleep. Pressure areas need most careful attention. For bedmaking, the child should be lifted rather than rolled from side to side so as to keep the intraperitoneal fluid localized. The upright position is adopted for the same reason and at the same time this will encourage deep respirations. Warmth may relieve abdominal pain and rigidity. Open windows and the use of electric fans help to reduce hyperpyrexia. Fluid balance charts are kept, as well as 4-hourly temperature readings and accurate observation charts.

With the help of a stethoscope, the bowel sounds should be checked as the absence of peristalsis, flatus and bowel actions are signs of intestinal paralysis. A blood transfusion is sometimes given to correct anaemia.

At times the free fluid in the abdomen may fail to absorb and become infected. A generalized septicaemia may develop or, in more favourable cases, the pus will localize and form a pelvic abscess. Adhesions may form between the convolutions of the bowel and later give rise to colic and obstruction.

Subphrenic abscess

Rarely, the pus localizes below the diaphragm causing an abscess which is difficult to palpate and diagnose. Treatment is by surgical drainage.

Pelvic abscess

Pelvic abscess rarely requires surgical interference. The pus localizes and, in the majority of cases, the abscess eventually ruptures into the rectum. Pus and mucus are passed when the child has his bowels opened. This complication delays recovery by a week or two but is rarely very serious, although the child may have considerable pain.

Paralytic ileus

When the serious complication of paralytic ileus arises, peristalsis ceases and there is complete constipation; no flatus is passed and the abdomen is distended and resonant when tapped. Vomiting may be severe and continues even when the normal stomach contents have been vomited; the vomit consists only of gastric and intestinal secretions mixed with bile.

Treatment consists of resting the bowel completely until peristalsis is re-established. Continuous gastric suction, or frequent aspirations by syringe through a nasogastric tube are carried out until there is no more aspirate and bowel sounds can be heard through a stethoscope.

Fluids are given only by the intravenous route until peristalsis is once more present. The child will need a good deal of nursing attention. He is usually restless and needs comforting. Hands and face should be sponged from time to time; the mouth treated regularly; the position of the limb into which the infusion is running, adjusted and supported by small pillows and the hands restrained to prevent him from pulling out the aspiration tube. Thirst may be troublesome and occasionally it may be permissible to give very small, infrequent cubes of ice to suck. Once peristalsis has started again, recovery is rapid and the child is, as a rule, eager to have his meals; he gains strength rapidly. Initially, the introduction of oral fluids should be slow and as the condition improves the process may be speeded up by introduction of easily digested foods.

Appropriate antibiotics are prescribed according to the seriousness of the causative organism, determined by blood culture and from a swab of the discharging wound.

Mesenteric lymphadenitis

Children often complain of abdominal pain for which there is no obvious explanation. The pain is not usually severe and neither guarding nor tenderness on examination are marked. There may occasionally be vomiting. The condition resolves itself without treatment and recurs from time to time. Although the symptoms are unconvincing, laparotomy is sometimes performed in order to exclude acute or subacute appendicitis. It will then be seen that the mesenteric lymph nodes are enlarged. It is thought that the enlargement is due to a generalized reaction of lymph tissue to infection. The condition is not a serious one but because of the possibility of appendicitis or renal tract disease, it should never be taken lightly.

Hernia

A hernia is a protrusion of an organ from the cavity in which it is normally contained. The following describe two types of hernia commonly encountered in children.

Umbilical hernia

Umbilical hernia is a very common condition of childhood. It is entirely harmless, although it is unsightly, but may cause parents much worry and may be thought by them to be the cause of such disturbances as wind and colic. The defect consists of a small, oval-shaped weakness in the linea alba, through which a loop of gut protrudes, and in the majority of cases it disappears spontaneously during the first 3 or 4 years of life. Small umbilical hernias rarely call for treatment but larger ones resolve more rapidly if surgical treatment is given. This is a simple repair of the hernia and can be done as a minor operation as an outpatient or as a day case. Trusses, adhesive strapping and elastic bandages are useless.

Inguinal hernia

Inguinal hernias are due to a developmental weakness in the abdominal wall and are usually first seen when the child cries, strains at stool, or coughs (particularly during the paroxysms of whooping cough). A small lump appears just lateral to and above the crest of the pubic bone. Occasionally this lump spreads down into the scrotum. It usually disappears when the child is at rest, or if he is held with shoulder and head lower than the rest of the body. In the majority of cases, operation is the treatment of choice. The operation is a minor one, consisting of locating and excising the hernial sac; it can be carried out in an outpatients' theatre, or the child can be admitted as a day case. Postoperatively the child is allowed the freedom of the cot as soon as he feels like it, and he can be allowed up on the day after the operation.

Inguinal hernias occur more frequently in boys than in girls because in development before birth, or in some cases during infancy and early childhood, the testes migrate through the inguinal canals into the scrotum. There is therefore a certain weakness in the abdominal wall in boys due to the fact that the inguinal canal is patent and the track through which the testes descend has not become obliterated. If either of the testes remains undescended it has to be brought down into the scrotum by a surgical operation (orchidopexy). Often at operation for undescended testicles, a hernial sac is also found and herniotomy performed.

If an inguinal hernia is sufficiently large or the neck of the hernial sac very narrow, the hernia can become irreducible and there is a danger of intestinal obstruction. As the child draws up his legs in pain and cries, the abdominal pressure increases and so aggravates the state of affairs. A sedative should be given and the buttocks and foot end of the cot raised. Occasionally the child is put into a warm bath or is nursed in a gallows-type of extension. Alternatively an ice-bag is suspended over the area to reduce the engorgement caused by the constriction of vessels in the inguinal canal. As the child relaxes, gravity causes the intestinal loop to slip back into the abdominal cavity, and the hernia reduces itself. Once this kind of situation has arisen, operation and repair should be carried out at an early date. If the hernia cannot be reduced by any of these methods, an operation should be carried out before a strangulated hernia occurs, as if this happens the blood supply to the loop of the gut is cut off, and this leads to gangrene of the loop.

Jaundice

Jaundice is the yellow staining of the skin and conjunctiva of the eyes by pigments absorbed from the blood instead of being excreted in the bile, as in a healthy person. It is therefore a symptom and not a disease in itself and there are several causes, some of which are dealt with in the appropriate chapter in greater detail. Jaundice arises if the breakdown of red cells is so rapid that the liver cannot cope with it. The unconjugated bilirubin in the circulation then rises. If, in the case of babies, it exceeds the normal level of 340 μmol/litre (20 mg/100 ml) of blood, bilirubin will be deposited in the ganglia of the nervous system, resulting in spasticity and mental handicap. Low birthweight babies and those with haemolytic disease are at particular risk, and frequent estimations of the serum bilirubin levels have to be performed and appropriate treatment given when danger point is reached. The main causes of jaundice in childhood can be grouped under the following headings.

The haemolytic types

These are due to excess destruction of red cells, i.e. at a greater rate than the liver can deal with. As these bile pigments are not excreted by the kidneys but are eliminated by the liver, stools and urine retain their normal colour. Examples are:

1. Haemolytic disease of the newborn (see p. 57).
2. Acholuric jaundice (see p. 191).
3. Transfusion jaundice.

Obstructive jaundice

This is caused by an obstruction in the bile ducts so that bile pigment cannot reach the duodenum. Stools are pale or even colourless but the urine is heavily coloured, and the skin is tinged yellow to olive colour. Examples are:

1. Biliary atresia (see p. 234).
2. Obstruction from pressure of a tumour or a choledochus cyst.
3. Very rarely obstruction by gall-stones or roundworms.

Jaundice due to sepsis

The principal examples are infection spreading from the umbilicus of the newborn, or general infection spreading via the blood stream and causing liver damage. In these instances the jaundice is rarely very deep.

Infective or acute virus hepatitis

This type of jaundice frequently appears in epidemic form. Serum hepatitis comes under this heading and this is caused by contamination with virus-infected blood or needles used for injections and blood tests. The urine is dark while the faeces are pale or colourless. There is a similar neonatal 'giant cell' hepatitis.

Other conditions accompanied by jaundice are congenital syphilis, galactosaemia, cystic fibrosis of the pancreas, physiological jaundice and Weil's disease.

Congenital atresia of the bile duct

In spite of the fact that atresia of a bile duct is congenital, symptoms may be at first either missed or mistaken for physiological jaundice. Contrary to the jaundice in the physiological variety, the jaundice in the case of obliteration of the bile duct fails to improve and the baby becomes more deeply jaundiced until he is almost an olive colour. The urine and saliva are stained with bile, the stools are grey, clay coloured or white and the liver is enlarged and firm. The obstruction to the normal flow of bile is due to a complete block, or absence of a segment of the common bile duct, so that bile cannot pass through it.

Diagnostic laparotomy is performed to pinpoint the site of the atresia and to take a liver biopsy. If a gall bladder is present, a radio-opaque substance is injected and this will outline the anatomy of the biliary tract under X-ray (cholecystography).

If a bile duct of adequate size is present, surgery, which aims at anastomosing it to a loop of bowel, is performed. Complications commonly occurring are: breakdown of the anastomosis; leakage of bile and attendant excoriation of skin; and post-operative bleeding due to delayed clotting time, despite pre-operative cover with vitamin K.

If operation is not possible, the jaundice gradually

deepens, liver and spleen enlarge and cirrhosis of the liver develops. Death takes place within two years.

THE COLON, RECTUM AND ANUS

Megacolon

Megacolon means enlarged colon. It may be:

1. The result of chronic constipation.
2. Due to a narrowing of the rectum.
3. Caused by an absence of the parasympathetic ganglia of the rectum, e.g. as in Hirschsprung's disease.

The treatment of the first two causes may require initial manual evacuation of the rectum under general anaesthesia, and frequent rectal washouts using normal saline and aperients such as Senokot. These measures must be combined with toilet training to redevelop normal bowel habits. In cases where the megacolon is secondary to chronic constipation, the nurse should appreciate that there may also be present quite a severe degree of psychological disturbance, and the help of the psychiatrist may be needed.

Hirschsprung's disease

Hirschsprung's disease (Fig. 34) is due to the absence of the parasympathetic ganglia in the rectum and occasionally farther along the long intestine, perhaps even beyond the sigmoid colon. As peristaltic action is initiated and maintained by these nerve cells, normal bowel movements do not take place and the intestine above the affected part becomes grossly dilated, while the rectum is, as a rule, empty, smaller than usual and frequently in spasm.

The disease is present at birth, but delay in diagnosis may occur, depending on the length of the aganglionic segment. Constipation is the presenting symptom, and there is often a delay of passage of the first meconium stool, which in the

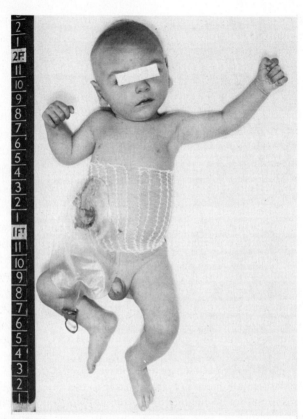

Fig. 34. Young infant with Hirschsprung's disease. Colostomy performed. Major surgery involving a radical pull through delayed until after the age of 6 months.

majority of normal babies is passed in the first 24 hours of birth.

Nursing management

Children with Hirschsprung's disease look miserable and unhappy, with thin wasted limbs in contrast to the big distended abdomen. The baby is often reluctant with his feeds and he will be inclined to vomit. As the condition progresses, visible peristalsis may be observed across the drum-like abdomen. Occasionally foul-smelling flatus and thin 'ribbon-like' stools are passed. Characteristic rumbling noises can be heard; these are known as borborygmi. At intervals the mucous lining of the bowel becomes inflamed and the stagnated, putrefied, offensive bowel content is passed. This enterocolitis can at first be mistaken for gastroenteritis and may rapidly lead to a dangerous loss of body fluids, requiring intravenous replacement. Characteristically, the distension and constipation may be relieved by digital examination of the rectum or by irrigation, and the child's condition will improve for a short period. Chest complications are common, as the distension of the abdomen impedes respiration by pressure on the diaphragm.

Babies suffering from Hirschsprung's disease cannot thrive unless treated, surgery being the only hope of survival. Commonly, if the affected segment is a relatively short one, the child will present at a later age as a failure to thrive, appearing puny and stunted in growth. It is through good nursing observations and reporting, that the lead to Hirschsprung's disease can often be given. Accurate recording of the number of bowel actions, and the nature of any stools passed, will bring abnormalities to the notice of medical staff at an early date. The putrefied smell often associated with bouts of diarrhoea, and the abdominal distension which causes the umbilicus to evert and the abdominal veins to be unusually prominent, are often first observed through daily handling and nursing care of the patient.

Barium enema

Diagnosis may be confirmed with the aid of a barium enema. When Hirschsprung's disease is suspected the normal pre-examination bowel preparation is omitted.

Rectal biopsy

A submucous biopsy is taken to demonstrate the absence of ganglion cells. This can now be obtained with a special instrument using suction, which avoids the need for general anaesthesia.

Anorectal manometry

This demonstrates the absence of the normal reflex inhibition of the internal anal sphincter on rectal distension, and is useful as a screening test.

Surgical management

Most commonly, Hirschsprung's disease is diagnosed as an emergency, the child presenting with acute symptoms and requiring immediate surgical intervention. A colostomy will be performed and surgery delayed until the child is 6–12 months old, or the symptoms have subsided.

The immediate pre-operative preparation is the same as for any other major abdominal operation. An intravenous infusion is set up, and a nasogastric tube passed.

Colostomy

General management of a colostomy in children differs little from that in an adult. In the immediate post-operative period there is danger of bleeding from the bowel and this is best stopped by the application of a firm bandage and a gauze pad soaked in a solution of adrenaline 1:1000. Occasionally the protruding bowel becomes strangulated and the opening in the abdominal wall has to be enlarged. A loop of bowel may prolapse through the incision and if this happens a pack of warm, sterile saline is applied until the patient can be taken back to the theatre. The delicate skin of children needs particularly careful attention. The surrounding area and buttocks should be washed frequently and no soiled pads left on longer than necessary. A barrier cream should be applied. The protruding bowel is protected from damage by a layer of tulle gras. If washouts are ordered they are done with a very soft catheter for fear of perforating the bowel.

With care the bowel can be regulated so as to produce a semi-formed stool which is easily passed but not too messy, and bowel actions can be reduced to twice daily. Extra nourishment and vitamins should be given, keeping in mind the fact that absorption can take place only in part of the length of the digestive tract.

The psychological aspect of a colostomy is of little importance in infants, but it is important to remember the effect such an operation may have on the mother. As a rule she can be reassured that the colostomy is merely a temporary measure. Permanent colostomy, performed for a congenital abnormality of the lower bowel, will of course cause greater distress to the parents and they will need a long period of adjustment and sympathetic support. Children with a permanent colostomy can be fitted with a colostomy belt and a normal life should be possible.

Surgical correction

The two most common operative procedures for Hirschsprung's disease are Swenson's (Fig. 35) and Duhamel's (Fig. 36) operations. Each involves laparotomy, mobilization of bowel, resection and reconstitution of the lower alimentary tract and often a temporary colostomy for the post-operative period.

Prior to operation a course of phthalysulphathiazole is given to sterilize the bowel. Any anaemia is treated and blood is taken for grouping. The immediate pre-operative preparation is the same as for any other major operation. An intravenous infusion is set up, and a nasogastric tube passed.

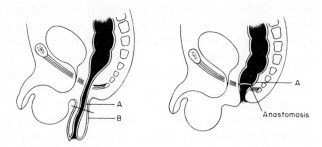

Fig. 35. Swenson's operation. *Left*: **The colon is mobilized, the rectum prolapsed through the anus allows an anastomosis.** *Right*: **Completion of the operation with the bowel returned to the pelvis, the ganglionic bowel (A) is anatomosed to the rectal stump.**

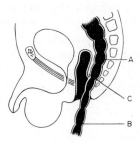

Fig. 36. Duhamel operation. Aganglionic bowel (B) is pulled down behind the closed rectum through the internal sphincter until the normally innervated bowel (A) is pulled through and fixed to the distal rectum. The aganglionic section that is pulled through is excised and the spur (C) is crushed with a clamp applied at the end of the operation.

Post-operative management

Intravenous therapy will be needed for the first 24 hours or so, as the child will be allowed nothing by mouth. During this time careful mouth toilet will be required to keep the mouth moist. Frequent observations must be recorded including a quarter-hourly pulse rate. If the pulse rate is rising a doctor should be informed, as in Hirschsprung's disease this is often a sign of fluid loss from an inflamed bowel. A nasogastric tube will be in position and should be aspirated 1–2-hourly. Providing the amount of aspirate is low and bowel sounds are heard, feeding with clear fluids can be commenced 24–48 hours after operation. The intravenous infusion can then be discontinued. Gradually, over the next few days, a normal diet is introduced.

The perianal skin may become sore, and should be washed frequently and a barrier cream applied. As the child's condition improves ambulation can be encouraged. Sutures are removed at about the eighth post-operative day if the wound is well healed. The colostomy is cared for and is closed about 2 weeks later.

Prognosis is excellent for these children. Regular bowel training is necessary at first. The mother is taught to give her child an adequate intake of roughage and fluids to avoid constipation. Occasional laxative may be required.

Rectal prolapse

When a section of mucous membrane comes down and presents at the anal orifice, the condition is known as rectal prolapse. Only rarely do all the coats of the rectum come down in this way and if this happens the condition is called *rectal procidentia*.

Rectal prolapse is a common occurrence in children of about 9 months to 3 years. There are several underlying causes and each will have to be treated before improvement can be expected from either medical or surgical therapy. The following are the usual causes: poor muscle tone, as in diseases of the nervous system; malnutrition and wasting disease, in which the supporting fatty tissue is absent; stress from coughing, as in whooping cough; long-standing diarrhoea causing irritation of the lower bowel; general mismanagement; behaviour problems; poor toilet training, long periods spent sitting on the pot; and finally mental handicap.

Nursing management

When a rectal prolapse occurs it should be dealt with calmly and the prolapse gently reduced. In most cases it can easily be pushed back by steady pressure with a piece of damp cotton wool while the patient is lying on his back. Alternatively, very young children can be held up by their legs when gravity may cause the prolapse to reduce itself. It may help if, after reducing the prolapse, the nurse holds the child's buttocks together for a few minutes, while she distracts his attention by telling a story or playing with him.

Patients who have had prolapses over a long period of time may have to learn to defaecate in a recumbent position. Sometimes a small toilet seat can be fixed over the adult lavatory to avoid the child adopting a squatting position. Good, consistent toilet training is a very important part of the treatment, but young children should not be allowed to sit on their pots for long, nor should undue importance be attached to a daily bowel action. A day or two missed will rarely be of consequence and is preferable to fussing over this point.

Surgical intervention is rare and occurs in intractable or long-standing cases. There is no pre-operative treatment although some surgeons may order a rectal washout before the patient is sent to the theatre. Post-operatively, the buttocks may be strapped together for 4 or 5 days. Extra fluids, a roughage free diet and liquid paraffin are given, to ensure soft stools and easy bowel action without straining.

Anal stenosis

Some babies are born with anal stenosis. This abnormality is not recognized on first examination but the baby will pass toothpaste-like stools and will be seen to strain at defaecation. Treatment consists in performing dilatations and giving laxative drugs.

According to the abnormality, signs and symptoms will

vary. If the condition is missed, the three typical signs of obstruction, vomiting, abdominal distension, and complete constipation, will develop in the case of severe stenosis or absence of an anal opening. If there is a moderate degree of stenosis, stools are passed but they are shaped like tooth-paste and the baby will strain on defaecation. If the anal opening is displaced, meconium will appear in an abnormal position.

Diagnosis

Diagnosis is made by thorough inspection, by digital examination and by radiographs. The baby is held upside down under the X-ray screen and this causes intestinal gases to rise to the apex of the blind pouch. A marker is placed over the anal dimple and the distance between this and the apex is measured. In this way a concise diagnosis can be made and the distance between the blind end of bowel and the perineum can be determined.

Treatment

Treatment depends on the type of abnormality. Very briefly, anal stenosis is treated by dilatation and laxatives; hidden anus with normal rectum, by incision of the covering membrane and dilatation; anal opening on the perineum but in a forward displaced position, by incision of the perineum and stitching of rectal mucosa round the new opening, followed by dilatation over a period of months. Recto-urethral and rectovaginal fistulae require major surgery and the creation of temporary or permanent colostomy (see p. 234).

Imperforate anus

During the first examination of the newborn baby, careful inspection of the perineum must always be included. Fail-ure of the baby to pass meconium must always arouse suspicion that an abnormality of the anus is present. The deformity may be superficial or deep. The anus may merely be hidden by skin which covers a normal rectum and sphincter, or the opening of the anal canal may be displaced forward on the perineum. In more severe deformities the rectum forms a fistula, which in the male communicates with the urethra and in the female with the vagina, there being a gap between the anal dimple seen on the perineum and the blind end of the bowel. Surgical repair is usually attempted.

Further reading

HARRIES, J. T. (1977) *Essentials of Paediatric Gastroenterology*. London: Churchill Livingstone.

HARRIS, F. (1972) *Paediatric Fluid Balance*. Oxford: Blackwell Scientific.

JOLLY, H. (1981) *Diseases of Children*, 4th edn. Oxford: Blackwell Scientific.

MCLAREN, D. S. & BURMAN, D. (1982) *Textbook of Paediatric Nutrition*, 2nd edn. London: Churchill Livingstone.

MOWAT, A. P. (1979) *Liver Disorders in Childhood*. London: Butterworth.

ROY, C. C. (1975) *Paediatric Clinical Gastroenterology*, 2nd edn. St. Louis: C. V. Mosby.

WALKER-SMITH, J. (1979) *Diseases of the Small Intestine in Childhood*, 2nd edn. London: Pitman Medical.

YOUNG, D. & WELLER, B. F. (1979) *Baby Surgery*. London: Harvey, Miller & Medcalf.

10 Metabolism and absorption

Metabolic disorders should be suspected when there is mental handicap, abnormal hair or skin texture or colour, abnormal urine output or colour, excessive thirst, abnormal appetite and failure to grow. With such conditions, the urine and the blood should be examined. Special biochemical tests can be carried out. A number of these diseases originate from an absence or abnormality of an enzyme which is essential for a particular metabolic process.

RICKETS

Rickets occur as a result of lack of fat-soluble vitamin D in the diet and from lack of sunshine. Calcium and phosphorus metabolism fail, and serious, typical signs and symptoms occur.

Improved standards of living and nutrition, and a well-developed welfare service have caused rickets—once known as the English disease—to become rare amongst the indigenous population in the British population. The disease is seen amongst immigrant families, particularly Asian families, where the vitamin content of the traditional diet is often low, and may even be negligible if strict vegetarianism is adhered to.

Prevention

1. A well-balanced diet with vitamin supplements up to the age of 5 years.

2. As much time as possible spent in the sunlight. Exposure of the baby's cheeks to sunlight for even a few hours is said to be sufficient for a day's requirement of vitamin D.

3. Cooperation between doctors, midwives, health visitors, teachers and nurses to identify children at risk and those showing early signs of tiredness, pain and weakness in the lower limbs and often with a poor posture. Emphasis on the value of sunlight and vitamin supplements should be made to newly arrived Asian immigrant families, with the help of the local community leaders and translators to overcome any language problem.

Active rickets

The groups at risk are infants, toddlers and young adolescents. It is caused by lack of vitamin D, which is essential for the utilization of calcium and phosphorus for good bone growth. Neither human nor cow's milk provide sufficient vitamin D for the baby's needs after the first weeks of life. The deficiency may also be produced by prematurity, lack of exposure to sunshine, faulty diet and inability to absorb the fat-soluble vitamin D in diseases such as coeliac disease. The risk period for vitamin D deficiency is during the winter, especially in northern cities where the daylight hours are shorter than in the south.

Signs and symptoms

In severe cases, the entire bony system of the body can be involved. The sutures and fontanelles of the skull are late in closing and together with bossing of the forehead give the skull the so-called 'hot cross bun' effect. Thinning of the cranial bones causes a resilience known as *craniotabes*. Dentition is delayed and the teeth are defective. The affected infant sits up and walks late, the bones are soft, arms and legs are bent and the epiphyses are enlarged. Respiration causes sucking in of the softened ribs, which results in a horizontal groove, known as *Harrison's sulcus*,

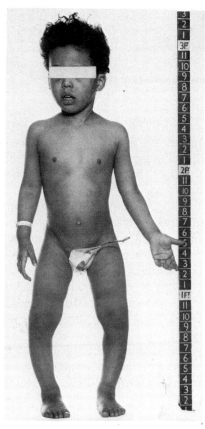

Fig. 37. A child with well-developed rickets. Urine bag in position for collection of specimen.

running round the anterior aspect of the chest. At the same time, beading at the juncture of the ribs and sternal cartilages forms the *rickety rosary*. The pelvic bones may become flattened and the angle of the neck of the femur on its shaft alters and eventually leads to limping, and in girls to obstetric complications in later life.

The abdomen in children with rickets is protuberant and there is a tendency to respiratory tract infections, sweating, diarrhoea and vomiting. The child is often miserable and sleeps little. Tetany, carpopedal spasm and laryngismus stridulus are all now rare complications.

Treatment

This consists of giving adequate amounts of vitamin D and minerals in the diet, which should be rich in milk, butter, fortified margarine, fresh eggs, green vegetables, meat and oily fish. This will require adjusting according to religious dietary laws.

The diet should be supplemented by vitamin D concentrates. Daily doses of 5000–50 000 iu (international units) of vitamin D or of calciferol by intramuscular injection or by mouth may be ordered in the active, acute stage.

The wearing of thick napkins should be avoided as they may cause bowing of the femora by holding the legs apart. Deformities are prevented by restricting walking and crawling in the acute stages and by nursing the infant on a firm, flat mattress.

Advice and education should be given to the parents to prevent recurrence of the disease and to protect the remaining members of the family. The health visitor and general practitioner will be able to provide local support.

PHENYLKETONURIA

Phenylketonuria is an inherited metabolic disorder, in which there is a failure to metabolize the amino acid, phenylalanine. This is due to the absence of the liver enzyme, phenylalaninase.

The majority of children with phenylketonuria are fair, with blue eyes, a marked tendency to eczema, a small head, large alveolar arches and widely spaced teeth. Their growth is stunted and they are late in sitting up. There is a peculiar musty odour to the urine of these children and they often suffer from epileptic fits.

The basis of treatment lies in the dietary limitation of phenylalanine. Some of this essential amino acid must be given for normal tissue growth and repair, but not enough for an abnormal accumulation to develop in the blood. For treatment to be effective it must commence between the age of 2–6 weeks. Therefore, the early detection of phenyl-ketonuria is of utmost importance if mental handicap is to be prevented.

The Guthrie test

A drop of blood is taken from a heel prick direct onto a filter paper and sent to the laboratory for specific culture tests, which will show whether there is an increased level of phenylalanine in the blood. The normal phenylalanine level is 0.06–0.12 mmol/litre (1–2 mg/100 ml).

The test is reliable after the first week of life.

The diet

The basis of treatment lies in the dietary limitation of phenylalanine. Some of this essential amino acid must be given for normal tissue growth and repair, but not enough for an abnormal accumulation to develop in the blood.

Infants. Human milk is lower in protein and phenylalanine per unit of nitrogen than cow's milk. A 15% solution of Minafen (Cow & Gate) before each breast-feed lowers the intake of protein and phenylalanine by reducing the amount of breast milk taken.

Small amounts of cereal can be started at 3–4 months. Reduced protein foods are not introduced until breast-feeding is discontinued.

Older children. Aminogran (Allen & Hanbury's). The changeover from Minafen/breast milk to Aminogran should be made slowly. Ketovite vitamin supplements are essential to maintain health.

Successful treatment is monitored by maintaining dietary treatment according to serum phenylalanine levels, below 0.03 mmol/litre.

GALACTOSAEMIA

Galactosaemia is a familial disease caused by an inability to metabolize galactose and so leading to intoxication of the body and brain cells. The result is mental deficiency, cataract and cirrhosis of the liver. The baby fails to thrive, is drowsy, refuses his feed and vomits. Jaundice may be present from the first day of life. Oedema may give a false impression of a satisfactory gain in weight. The stools are loose and the liver becomes enlarged.

Treatment

Treatment must be started at once if it is to be effective. It entails substituting all feeds containing galactose or lactose by special preparations such as Nutramigen or Galactomin. Where these are not available, soya bean 'milk' to which Casilan, cane sugar, coconut oil, minerals and vitamins can be added, may be given.

Diagnosis

Whenever there is a familial history of the disease a simple test can be carried out on the cord blood, or alternatively a urine test will show the presence of galactosuria. Any finding of sugar in the urine must always be reported at once so that more specialized laboratory tests can be carried out. It is important to note that testing with the usual reagents will show sugar present in the urine, as the reaction is due to glucose.

DISORDERS OF LIPOID AND GLYCOGEN STORAGE

This group of diseases includes such rare conditions as xanthomatosis, Schüller-Christian syndrome, Gaucher's disease, Niemann-Pick disease and lipoidosis. In the last, abnormal amounts of various lipoids are stored in the reticulo-endothelial system. The chief damage is in the brain cells, but in spite of this, diagnosis can be confirmed by a simple rectal biopsy involving approximately 1 cm of full thickness bowel wall.

HYPOGAMMAGLOBULINAEMIA (IMMUNODEFICIENCY DISEASE)

Hypogammaglobulinaemia is a rare condition mostly seen in boys and the principal manifestation is a marked tendency to infections, as the lack of gamma globulin prevents antibody formation.

Treatment

Gamma globulin is given by weekly injections and in some cases prophylactic antibiotic treatment is ordered. Where a suitable donor can be found, bone marrow transfusion is given. This, combined with reverse barrier nursing in the initial phase of the disease, offers the best hope of a normal life.

STEATORRHOEA

Steatorrhoea is a symptom rather than a disease in itself and is the passage of fluid or excessively soft stools containing an unusual amount of fat.

Steatorrhoea may be caused by some disturbance in the function of the small intestine and the amount of fat present in the stools may vary from amounts so small that they are only found in the process of careful analysis, to visible, oily globules on the surface of the stools.

Signs and symptoms

The stools have a characteristic, highly offensive smell. Their appearance is putty-coloured, unformed and bulky and their frothy quality suggests the presence of fermentation. Occasionally fatty globules can be seen on the surface. The frequent loose evacuations may alternate with periods of constipation. Abdominal distension, redness around the anus, excoriated buttocks and rectal prolapse often accompany the steatorrhoea.

The affected child fails to thrive.

The abnormal fat losses and frequent stools may cause secondary symptoms such as a voracious appetite and tetany due to loss of calcium, which in turn results in a low blood calcium level, dehydration, stunted growth and lassitude.

Investigations

Investigations depend on the suspected, underlying cause and may include:

Mantoux test and X-ray of abdomen (tuberculosis).

Barium meal and X-ray (congenital abnormalities affecting the gut).

Glucose tolerance curve (this is flat in coeliac disease).

Analysis of duodenal secretions and stools for tryptic activity (fibrocystic disease of the pancreas).

Sweat tests.

Examination of stools for ova, cysts, starch granules and excess of fat.

A fat balance may be done as one of the investigations.

3-day stool collection for fat content estimation.

Stool collection for fat estimation. The simplest form of faecal fat estimation is carried out on stools collected over three consecutive days. The normal excretion being 5 g of fat in a 24-hour period, the excess is estimated. If a more accurate estimation is required an estimation of the amount ingested against that excreted is calculated.

All faeces must be collected and it is useful to line nappies or bedpans with cellophane or plastic material during the test period. The faeces can then be easily lifted into the collecting receptacle.

COELIAC DISEASE

Coeliac disease is a chronic condition which is commonly diagnosed during childhood, usually at the age of weaning.

The disease is caused by malabsorption of food from the intestines and there is an abnormal sensitivity to gluten, found in wheat and rye.

Signs and symptoms

Children with coeliac syndrome are stunted in growth and underweight and X-ray examination reveals osteoporosis (rarefaction) and immature development of bone due to poor vitamin absorption and calcium deficiency. Excess gas formation caused by fermentation of malabsorbed food causes abdominal pain and vomiting. The patient has a large, protuberant abdomen. The buttocks are wasted and the skin hangs in loose folds. The stools are bulky, putty coloured, unformed and greasy and have a characteristic, putrefied smell. The child may have his bowels opened several times a day.

The child himself looks frail, stunted, pale and wizened, and usually utterly miserable, though the face may at first look round and well. The hair is sparse and dry, the limbs thin as drumsticks and cold to the touch. Poor muscle tone reflects itself in bad posture and rectal prolapse is common. Anaemia is a usual feature. The appetite is very poor and capricious. These children often have the strangest whims and their feeding may tax the ingenuity and patience of the nurse and his parents to the utmost.

Investigations

Analysis of stools, i.e. fat content, a complete blood count, a glucose tolerance test, a xylose excretion test and jejunal biopsy may all be performed. The jejunal biopsy is done with the aid of a Crosby capsule (Fig. 38) and may reveal characteristic flatness of the mucosa of duodenum and jejunum.

Jejunal biopsy. The child is starved for 4–6 hours before the procedure commences. Sedation may be prescribed. The doctor usually passes the Crosby capsule into the stomach. Gastric movement and peristaltic movement passes the capsule into the duodenum. With the aid of radiographs to ensure the capsule is in the jejunum, the capsule is 'fired'. The capsule is withdrawn containing the biopsy specimen of intestinal mucosa.

Following completion of the biopsy, the child is allowed to rest 12–24 hours. The child is observed for signs of haemorrhage or perforation. Diet is gradually reintroduced over a 24-hour period, providing complications of perforation and haemorrhage do not occur.

Nursing management

Admission to hospital cannot always be avoided, but the stay should be cut to a minimum while investigations are carried out, diagnosis confirmed and treatment established. Occasionally these children are acutely ill and during that time require more intensive nursing care.

Because of weight loss and emaciation, skin and mouth require special attention. Mouth toilet is carried out frequently and pressure areas treated 2–4-hourly. Crumbs,

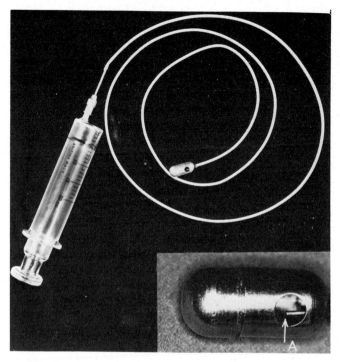

Fig. 38. A Crosby capsule, used to obtain small specimens of intestinal mucosa. (A) Mechanism fired to obtain specimen of intestinal mucosa.

wrinkled or damp sheets are avoided to prevent pressure sores, which will not heal easily. After a bath the skin should be dried carefully, and the child should not be left sitting on a pot or bedpan for longer than necessary.

As soon as possible, these children should be allowed to get up and lead a normal life. Schooling or play therapy are important in stimulating interest and speedy recovery. Frequent visiting will not only help the young patient but will also teach the mother much about the handling of her child and about the special diet.

Diet

The main treatment is the introduction of a diet which is free of gluten, which is contained in wheat and rye. Gluten-free bread, cakes and rusks can be obtained and gluten-free flour is available to make into cakes, bread, biscuits and puddings. Lists of proprietary foods that are gluten free is available from a dietician. At first, the fat content of the diet may be restricted and extra protein added. However, if all foods containing wheat and rye are omitted, a normal amount of fat can soon be taken.

A satisfactory diet can be given, without much extra work, if foods made of maize (corn), oats, rice, sago, and tapioca (not semolina) are substituted for those made of wheat and rye. Extra vitamin A and D, folic acid and iron should be given.

The diet is continued for life, although small amounts of gluten may be tolerated as the child grows and becomes an adult. Gluten should be avoided during at least the first 2–5 years after diagnosis. The mother should be told that even minor deviations from the prescribed diet in the early stages of the disease may cause serious relapse.

Prognosis

The improvement is rapid following introduction of the diet. The stools soon become less bulky and offensive, the appetite improves and the child gains weight and is happier. Provided care is taken with the diet, this improvement should be maintained.

Complications

Complications include intercurrent infections; oedema due to low serum protein; rickets and tetany due to impaired absorption of the fat-soluble vitamins.

As excess amounts of potassium and fluids are lost in the large stools, 'coeliac crises' due to electrolyte depletion occasionally call for urgent action. The child suddenly becomes severely dehydrated, lethargic and collapses. The temperature may rise by several degrees. Intravenous therapy may be necessary to correct both the blood chemistry and the dehydration.

CYSTIC FIBROSIS (MUCOVISCIDOSIS)

This condition is characterized by a disturbance of exocrine gland function, resulting in raised levels of sodium chloride in the sweat and thick mucous secretions from the secretory glands. In this country it is the most common of the inborn errors of metabolism, with an incidence of 1 in 2000 births. More than one child in the family may be affected as the disease is transmitted as a recessive gene carried by each parent.

The production of the abnormal mucus results in chronic lung infections, pancreatic insufficiency and intestinal obstruction in the newborn (meconium ileus).

Signs and symptoms

Unlike the child suffering from coeliac disease, children with cystic fibrosis are friendly and good tempered. The appetite remains good in the absence of general infection but in spite of this there is failure to gain weight, growth is stunted, the abdomen is distended giving the child a 'barrel-like' appearance. The stools are pale and bulky, bowel actions are frequent and the smell is characteristically offensive.

When the disease is well-established at birth, intestinal obstruction results due to the failure to pass meconium. This is because the enzyme which would normally liquefy the meconium is absent. This serious condition requires urgent treatment either by surgery or treatment by Gastrografin enema under X-ray control.

Repeated chest infections is often a presenting symptom, the gastrointestinal symptoms being revealed in the history.

Specific investigations

Boehringer meconium strip is smeared evenly with meconium and placed in water. Cystic fibrosis is diagnosed by the appearance of a bright blue colour at the end of the strip.

Sweat test is carried out simply, in outpatients, by placing the child's washed fingers on an agar plate containing silver nitrate and potassium chromate. In cystic fibrosis the excess of chlorides in the sweat show up by the fingerprint impression being grey. For a more accurate test a sample of sweat may be collected on a weighted piece of filter paper (free from sodium chloride) after inducing local sweating with pilocarpine iontophoresis. The filter paper is handled with forceps and taken to the laboratory in a sealed container for chemical analysis. A child with cystic fibrosis usually excretes more than 60 mmol of sodium chloride per litre.

Duodenal intubation allows specimens of duodenal juice (including pancreatic enzymes) to be aspirated and analysed. The child is starved for 4 hours prior to the procedure and a Ryle's tube is passed. The child lies in a right lateral position and gastric motility and peristaltic action conveys the tube into the pyloric sphincter and into the duodenum. The location of the tube in the duodenum can be made by noting the change from an acid to an alkaline reaction.

Tryptic activity is examined in specimens of faeces. Trypsin is a proteolytic enzyme which is one of the pancreatic enzymes which may be absent or diminished in cystic fibrosis.

Nursing management and treatment

Nursing action	Explanation
Pancreatic enzyme preparations are prescribed to be taken with all meals.	To replace the enzymes blocked in the pancreas.
Care to prevent irritation of the skin around the mouth.	The enzymes are strongly alkaline.
Reduced fat content in diet.	Medium chain triglyceride fats are more easily digested.
Vitamin supplements.	In particular, fat-soluble vitamin deficiencies are likely to occur.
Supplementary salt, particularly in hot climates.	Excessive sweating with high salt content is characteristic of the disease.
Chest physiotherapy with postural drainage and percussion. Parents are taught how to carry this out.	To clear the lungs of the thick tenacious mucus. Will be required for the rest of child's life.
Humidification of air breathed.	Helps to erase expectoration.
Prevention of cross-infection. Nurse away from children with other infections.	Poor lung drainage makes child susceptible to infection.
Frequent baths and changes of clothes.	Because of excessive sweating will promote patient's comfort and coolness.
Careful explanation to parents. Genetic counselling.	The disease is inherited by recessive genes.
Suggest the help and services of the medical socialworker. Alert parents to Cystic Fibrosis Society.	Social and emotional problems may arise. Contact with other families in the society will provide on-going support.
The health visitor and school nurse are informed of discharge.	To continue management and support at home.

During recent years, the prognosis of children with cystic fibrosis has much improved as a result of vigorous treatment and care to combat respiratory infections, which in the past have resulted in early death.

Further reading

ANDERSON, C. M. & GOODCHILD, M. C. (1976) *Cystic Fibrosis*. London: Blackwell Scientific.

FRANCIS, D. E. M. (1974) *Diets for Sick Children*, 3rd edn. London: Blackwell Scientific.

HOLTON, S. & TYFIELD, L. (1980) *The Child with Phenylketonuria*. West Yorkshire: NSPKU.

SINCLAIR, L. (1979) *Metabolic Disease in Childhood*. London: Blackwell Scientific.

11 The endocrine system

Diseases of the endocrine system are comparatively rare in childhood but when they occur they may have a serious effect on mental and physical growth and maturation.

THE THYROID GLAND

Thyrotoxicosis

Over-secretion, causing thyrotoxicosis, is very uncommon in childhood. If it occurs, methyl thiouracil, carbimazole or potassium perchlorate and very occasionally surgery are employed in its treatment, in much the same way as for adults.

Hypothyroidism

Under-secretion of the thyroid gland causes cretinism in children. The condition, though congenital, is sometimes missed at birth as the infant carries a small amount of thyroid secretion from the maternal circulation. As the amount decreases, general metabolism is slowed down and symptoms appear.

Signs and symptoms

All cretins have certain, typical characteristics. Their skin is cold, coarse and dry with a yellow appearance. The hair is brittle, sparse and lacks lustre and the hair line grows low down on to the constantly puckered brow. A broad, flat nose with a depressed bridge lies between the small widely spaced eyes. The lips are thick and as the tongue is apparently too large for the mouth, it protrudes. The abdomen is large, and constipation and umbilical hernia are common features. Pads of fat over the clavicles make the neck appear short. As bony development is retarded, the fontanelles are late in closing, the head seems disproportionately large and the first teeth are late in coming through. The entire appearance is heavy, coarse and dull. As general metabolism is suppressed, the temperature is subnormal and the pulse rate slow. Anaemia is common. Speech develops late and some achieve only an elementary vocabulary. The voice is croaky and unmelodious. All milestones are late and, if left untreated, the child will be severely mentally handicapped.

Although not all these characteristics are noticeable at birth, the nurse may first notice the umbilical hernia and the constipation and, if she is alert and well-informed, may link these symptoms with the low temperature and sluggish pulse. Most are poor feeders, at least partly due to the abnormally large tongue which makes sucking difficult and also causes attacks of suffocation. An observant nurse or midwife can contribute greatly to a good prognosis as early treatment is the key to success.

Investigations

The ones likely to be carried out are: blood cholesterol and serum lipid levels, both of which tend to be raised; creatinine and protein-bound iodine levels, which are abnormally low; X-ray of bones to estimate the bone age; electrocardiogram and blood picture. The basal metabolic rate is difficult to estimate in children but, if done, shows readings much below the normal.

Treatment

Treatment should be started without delay and will have

to be continued throughout life in order to replace the thyroxine which the abnormal gland cannot produce. Treatment may be so successful that the child develops normally. However, a great deal depends on the age at which treatment is begun. The treatment consists of giving thyroxine in dosages just below the point at which signs of intolerance appear. The initial dose for infants is 25 μg daily and this is increased until tachycardia, diarrhoea and wakefulness suggest that the dosage has passed the tolerance level. Tolerance may be higher during the cold season than in the summer months. The maintenance dose is fixed slightly below the maximum reached during the stabilizing period.

Nursing care and observations

During the initial stage, nursing care is symptomatic. The infant should be kept warm and the nurse feeding the baby will have to be both experienced and very patient. Suppositories or Milk of Magnesia will have to be given for the constipation and the skin should be kept supple with baby creams or lotions. Care must be taken when the baby is placed in his cot and it is safest to lie him on his side to guard against the danger of respiratory obstruction caused by the large tongue.

Once thyroid therapy has been started, the nursing observations will be the principal guide in determining the maintenance dosage. Signs of response, such as an increased pulse rate and a rise in the body temperature, are all due to an increase in the metabolic rate. There is an improvement in the infant's colour and activity and a drop in weight due to the disappearance of the excess fat. The bowels will start to act regularly. The infant will begin to look around and play and will become more interested in his feeds.

The nurse should keep full and accurate observation charts. The feeds may have to be large for a time to satisfy the newly found appetite and to supply adequate nourishment for the sudden progress. It is well worth while to arrange for a little extra attention by the mother or nurse to encourage every attempt at play and to help the infant develop his activities and mental achievements.

THE PITUITARY GLAND

The chief importance of the pituitary gland is probably its influence on the other ductless glands. Abnormalities of the anterior lobe cause gigantism if there is over-secretion, dwarfism if there is under-secretion. Abnormalities of the posterior lobe cause diabetes insipidus.

The abnormalities may be congenital or may be caused by pressure from intracranial tumours or by inflammatory conditions such as encephalitis. None of these conditions are sufficiently common to warrant description in a small handbook and the reader is referred to larger text books for greater detail.

The hormone activity of the gland, however, is of great interest. The pituitary gland produces adrenocortico-trophic hormone (ACTH) which makes the adrenal cortex produce hormones with three effects:

1. On carbohydrate metabolism.
2. On mineral metabolism affecting blood electrolytes.
3. On growth and maturity, including masculinization if there is excess in the female.

Growth hormone deficiency

Some children fail to grow normally, even though they were of normal weight and length at birth and the parents are known to be of average height and build. This type of growth failure is commonly due to deficient secretion of growth hormone from the anterior lobe of the pituitary.

Replacement therapy can be given by regular intramuscular injections of human growth hormone, usually over a period of 2–3 years at a specialized referral growth clinic.

THE ADRENAL GLANDS

Diseases of the adrenal and suprarenal glands are extremely rare in childhood and are usually due to tumours, injury at birth resulting in haemorrhage, or infections such as tuberculosis. Both the diagnosis and treatment are difficult, though the discovery of cortisone has contributed much to the understanding of the diseases caused by over- or under-secretion of the glands.

Tumours of the medulla are often malignant and cause metastases in the liver, lungs and bone tissue. Surgery in the less malignant type of tumours, however, carries a hopeful prognosis. The adrenal medulla produces adrenaline and noradrenaline which, like cortisone, have a place in the treatment of asthma and shock.

Over-activity of the adrenal cortex leads to sexual precocity in both sexes and to virilism in the female. The over-activity may be present before birth and in this case causes pseudohermaphroditism (see below). In the young child over-activity causes sexual precocity and virilism and if the anterior pituitary gland is secondarily affected, Cushing's syndrome will result. True Cushing's syndrome is rare in childhood but is often simulated when a child is having too large a dose of steroids. The child characteristically becomes 'moon-faced', looking flushed and bloated. Obesity develops, with pads of fat accumulating on the upper part of the back, producing a 'buffalo hump' together with a fat abdomen and hips. In contrast the limbs remain thin. Growth of hair occurs on the face and body, together with purple striae on the trunk. Acne is common. Hypertension is usually present, and the child may complain of headaches. Glycosuria may also be found on routine ward testing.

Adrenogenital syndrome

Very occasionally in some children there is difficulty in determining the sex of the child, owing to the malformation of the external genitalia in the male or masculinization of the genitalia in the female. This occurs as a congenital or as an acquired disorder. For a correct sex determination to be made it is necessary for chromosome studies to be carried out. To avoid distress to the parents and to the child in subsequent development it is important, in all these cases, that necessary examination of the blood, urine and smears from the buccal membrane are undertaken before the birth is registered.

Great understanding and tact is needed in helping the parents to understand and adjust to the condition of their child. Cortisone therapy and plastic surgery may be beneficial to some of these children. Nurses should see to it that these children are not subjected to unnecessary examinations as even very young children are sensitive to handling of the genital area.

Steroid therapy

The adrenal cortex produces hormones with three effects:

1. On carbohydrate metabolism.
2. On mineral metabolism affecting blood electrolytes.
3. On growth and maturity, including masculinization if there is excess in the female.

In addition, excessive amounts can damp down inflammatory reactions by interfering with antigen–antibody reactions and can cause the production of ACTH by the pituitary to be lowered.

Cortisone or similar preparations such as prednisone, prednisolone or triamcinolone can be given by mouth and hydrocortisone by injection for the following purposes:

1. To make up for deficiency of the adrenal activity as in shock or in Addison's disease.

2. To suppress the production of ACTH in cases of precocious sexual development of a masculine type.

3. To suppress antigen–antibody reaction, as in rheumatic fever, rheumatoid arthritis, some types of nephritis, asthma and haemolytic anaemia.

The use and choice of steroid depends upon the child's disease and condition, balanced against the known adverse effects of steroid therapy (see Table 6).

Long-term treatment

When long-term corticosteroid therapy is given, the maintainance dose should be kept as low as possible to minimize the side-effects. When treatment is to be discontinued, the dose should be reduced gradually over a period of several weeks.

The parents should be given a 'steroid card' giving details of dosage, together with the drug name and possible complications to be alert to. They should also know that if for any reason they need to seek other medical or dental care for their child the card should be presented to the practitioner before treatment is commenced. Anaesthetists also need to know if a child is taking or has been taking corticosteroids, as adrenal suppression may cause a precipitous fall in blood pressure during anaesthesia.

DIABETES MELLITUS

Children with diabetes suffer from deficient insulin action caused either by a diminished insulin excretion by the islets

Table 6. Adverse effects of steriod therapy and its management in children

Main adverse effects of steroid therapy in children	Due to	Nursing management
Weight gain Oedema Hypertension Disturbed electrolytes Tiredness Lethargy	The mineralocorticoid effect upon sodium and potassium metabolism	Daily weighing. Regular measurement of blood pressure. Maintain fluid record charts. Low salt diet
Suppression of growth	Excessive loss of calcium and phosphorus	Adequate calcium and protein in diet. Stunted growth may be mitigated by giving steroids only on alternate days
Glycosuria, which may lead to diabetes mellitus	Glucocorticoid effect on carbohydrate metabolism and insulin utilization	Daily urinalysis for glucose
May allow potentially very damaging infection to pass unrecognized, e.g. tuberculosis	Modification of tissue reaction resulting from suppression of antigen–antibody reaction	Keep child away from known infection. Be aware of risk and record child's temperature appropriately
Altered behaviour pattern		Note and report any change from usual behaviour

of Langerhans in the pancreas, or due to the presence of insulin antagonists which render any insulin produced ineffective for carbohydrate metabolism, resulting in glycosuria, ketosis and eventually coma.

Even newborn infants may occasionally suffer from diabetes, and apnoeic or cyanotic attacks in premature or ill-nourished infants should always be investigated. The disease, however, is very rare under the age of 2 years. In about a quarter of all cases there is a family history of diabetes.

In children, the onset of diabetes is usually very sudden and, although never actually responsible for the disease, infections such as tonsillitis or measles, and emotional stress seem to act as the trigger starting off the symptoms.

Signs and symptoms

Most obvious, and therefore often first noticed, is the sudden excessive thirst, coupled with frequency of micturition or the onset of enuresis in a previously clean child. The output of urine is large but in spite of this it is of high specific gravity. The child grows listless and fractious. As dehydration occurs, the skin becomes dry and he is constipated. The breath may smell of acetone. The tongue is dry but, as a rule, it remains clean but abnormally red. Loss of weight may be rapid and considerable and a proportion of children develop an unusual appetite.

The penis or vulva is often red and irritating due to the high sugar content of the urine, and the child may complain of abdominal pain. As ketosis increases, vomiting sets in and may hasten the occurrence of diabetic coma. The urine contains sugar and acetone.

Investigations

These include testing of urine, blood sugar estimation and glucose tolerance tests. Serum bicarbonate, blood pH and PCO will need estimating if ketoacidosis is present.

If possible, tests involving pricks and fasting should be spaced and not all done the first day after admission, as it is important to preserve the young patient's confidence since he will probably be starting on a lifetime of daily insulin injections.

Treatment

Some specialists like to treat these children as outpatients as they feel that the child should be assessed and stabilized under his usual living conditions. The majority feel, however, that the child should be admitted to hospital so that the investigations and the initial stabilizing can take place under controlled and known conditions. The fact that in hospital the child's activities are, of necessity, restricted should always be borne in mind. The mother should be asked about the child's normal routine, and exercise should be given so that the child's usual energy output is maintained.

Children with diabetes should never be kept in bed unnecessarily. From the start, a healthy attitude and interest should be fostered and any special diet should be accepted as a natural part of the young diabetic's routine.

It is essential that children with diabetes wear an identification bracelet or badge at all times.

The diet

With the present-day insulins, which are very stable and long-acting (e.g. the Lente group), the child, once stabilized, can be kept free from reactions by allowing his appetite to regulate his blood sugar levels. It will be found that if he has been unusually energetic he will also be very hungry, and if he has sat quietly for a time his appetite will decrease. Periodic tests to estimate the serum cholesterol levels are done. If the level rises, foods containing cholesterol are omitted from the diet (e.g. eggs) as a persistently raised serum cholesterol level predisposes to vascular changes in later life. Children receiving an unrestricted diet are much less likely to have psychological problems which children who are placed on a restricted diet tend to develop. However, some paediatricians continue to advocate a strictly controlled diet on the grounds that it lessens the chances of future vascular complications. For children who are learning about the importance of diet, playing cards, charts and games which help to memorize food values, exist. 'Rupert and his Friends' (Ames, Slough) is a useful booklet that can also be used as a teaching aid.

Insulin therapy

The dose of insulin will have to be readjusted until the condition is stabilized. This may not happen until some weeks after discharge home. Adjustment will usually become necessary when the child has an infection or any severe emotional upset; as he grows and increases in weight; and especially at the time of puberty. The aim is to find the dose which will enable the child to live a normal life on a diet adequate for growth, energy and enjoyment of life. It is here assumed that the reader has already a sound understanding of the types of insulin available and of the various syringes and their markings, as well as of the principles involved in insulin therapy. In these aspects there is no difference when dealing with young diabetics as compared with adults, but the approach to the problem of diabetes in childhood is important and specialized.

Both the parents and the child should be taught how to give injections and test the urine and, as far as they are capable, they should be taught to understand the principles involved. They should also be taught confidence and the child himself should take a healthy interest in his illness. By the age of 8 years it should be possible to teach a sensible

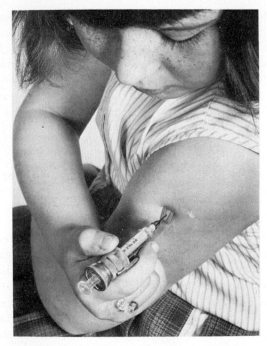

Fig. 39. Diabetic child giving own injection of insulin using automatic injector.

patient to give his own insulin and to draw up the dose himself, even if it is still checked by his parents (Fig. 39).

The site of the injections should be as varied as possible in order to prevent thickening of the tissues and local fat atrophy which, though harmless, causes unsightly depressions and irregularities in the contours of the limb. The injection should be given fairly deeply with the needle almost at right angles to the skin. Alternatively, a Palmer mechanical injector, shaped rather like a pistol, can be used.

General points

Both the young patient and his parents should be helped to come to grips with the disability and the latter should not be allowed to make the child into an invalid by misplaced solicitude. Both the parents and the child, once he is old enough, should be taught the fundamentals of the illness and should be allowed to practise urine testing and the giving of injections well before discharge, so as to gain confidence and dexterity in so doing.

It is a good plan to allow the child to experience one or more insulin reactions while still under supervision in hospital, so that after his discharge he will be able to guard himself in good time against any serious hypoglycaemic reaction.

N.B. It is planned, in the near future, to standardize on a single strength insulin of 100 units/ml (U100). This has the advantage of simplifying the measurement of dosages because it will be possible to read off the units of insulin directly on the U100 syringe. However, the choice between different insulin strengths remains (subject to their availability from the manufacturers) at least over the next few years (HN(82)32).

Education

Most diabetic children can attend normal schools provided the teachers know of their condition. Hypoglycaemic reaction is often heralded by naughty or unusual behaviour, and glucose or a lump of sugar may correct the hypoglycaemia without much disturbance. Teachers should have sugar or glucose available, but as soon as he is old enough the young diabetic should be made responsible for recognizing and dealing with a hypoglycaemic reaction by taking sugar from his own supply. It is possible to allow diabetic children to have the usual school meals, as the high carbohydrate content of school puddings supplies the extra amount needed during the exertion of the afternoon games period.

Holidays

Under controlled conditions and supervision, the Diabetic Association runs holiday camps which have the added value that the children meet other diabetics, often learn much from each other and come to realize that they are not alone with their abnormality.

Hyperglycaemic or diabetic coma

The signs of oncoming coma are essentially the same in children as in adults, but a child's behaviour may differ according to his age. Thus a very young child may demand to be put to bed or may curl up in a corner and fall asleep. Shock and dehydration often come on very rapidly and both may be severe.

Hypoglycaemic or insulin coma

Insulin coma comes on even more suddenly than diabetic coma. It often happens that the child is hard to wake in the morning and, when roused, looks pale and apprehensive and shows a peculiar emotional behaviour.

Points of importance

If there is any doubt about the nature of the reaction, the child should be given some glucose, as little harm can be done by hyperglycaemia, while insulin coma may require urgent relief. It is useful to remember that 2 slightly heaped teaspoonfuls of sugar in water equal approximately 10 g of carbohydrate.

Administering insulin—education of child and parents

Aim

The child with diabetes and at least one parent should be

fully competent in the preparing, drawing up and the giving of insulin.

Checklist

1. Do they all understand the need for insulin injections? Ask the parents, and the child where possible, for an explanation in their own words. Correct any misunderstandings. Provide with the literature that is available.

2. Provide syringe needles and opportunities to take these apart. Note their different pieces, structure and the measurements on the side of the barrel. Answer any questions fully.

3. Emphasize the need for cleanliness of hands, skin of injection site, and equipment for the prevention of any infection.

4. Discuss the need to rotate injection sites. Suggest it might be helpful for the child, initially, to keep a chart showing this rotation. The child may like to design one of his own, a decorated body outline is often a good idea.

5. Insulin. How this is obtained and the need to maintain supplies, and where to store vials, which should be in a cool place. Instruct carefully in the calculation of insulin dosage.

6. Finally, drawing up of the insulin and administering an injection. 'Try-outs' with sterile water on 'teddy' or oranges, or thick foam pads should be supervised. The giving of insulin under supervision is the final goal.

The assimilation of this new knowledge may take several days or weeks depending on many variable factors, e.g. age of the child, intelligence of the child and the parents, the impact of anxiety and stress impeding uptake of new knowledge. The nurse needs to be prepared to repeat each stage frequently and to reassure the child and the parents as to the progress being made. Set realistic goals for the family to achieve in realizing the aims set.

Further reading

BAILEY, J. D. (1982) *Paediatric Endocrinology*. London: W. B. Saunders.

BROOK, C. G. D. (1978) *Practical Paediatric endocrinology*. London: Academic Press.

DRURY, M. I. (1979) *Diabetes Mellitus*. Oxford: Blackwell Scientific.

FARQUHAR, J. W. (1981) *The Diabetic Child*, 3rd edn. London: Churchill Livingstone.

FARQUHAR, J. W. (1975) *Notes for the Guidance of Parents of Diabetic Children*, 2nd edn. London: Churchill Livingstone.

12 Problems of the nervous system and mental handicap

Basically, examination of a child's nervous system is the same as for an adult. A child, however, is unable to describe his symptoms accurately and he will often be irritable and uncooperative. It will always help if a nurse whom the child knows and trusts can be present to assist the paediatrician. It is important to allow plenty of time for the child to settle in the unfamiliar surroundings.

Most of the history of the child will be obtained from the mother and it is traced back to include information about pregnancy and delivery. It is important to know whether there were any signs of synosis or asphyxia at birth and whether the baby was pre-term or born at term. The paediatrician will also want to know if there is any family history of epilepsy, mental handicap or any other illness.

EXAMINATION OF THE NERVOUS SYSTEM

The paediatrician will note any abnormality of the skull such as bossing, asymmetry and the size of the fontanelles. In certain cases, such as suspected cerebral lesions or intercranial tumours, it may be important to notice the way in which the child holds his head.

The child may be unable to accurately reach objects held out to him or he may have a tremor of the hand. In certain diseases the way in which the child raises himself from the floor to a standing position is in itself diagnostic. Sometimes the absence or presence of normal skills gives the best guide towards assessment and diagnosis.

An assessment of the child's behaviour will be made in order to establish:

Motor development.
Activity patterns.
Speech development.
Cognitive development.
Sensory evaluation.

To test the reflexes is important. Reflexes in the very young infant are unusually brisk and the plantar reflex is still extensor and only becomes flexor, as in the adult, when the child starts to walk.

SOME NEUROLOGICAL PROCEDURES

Lumbar puncture

Lumbar puncture is the same for children as for adults and is done for the same reasons. Using a language which the child understands, he should be told simply why he needs to lie in an uncomfortable position for this procedure. An explanation should also be given to the parents. This will help to reassure the child and gain his cooperation. In some instances the mother may wish to be present and can sit by the child's head to comfort him. It is, however, important to have complete control of the child when holding him and only an experienced person should attempt to do this. Very young children are often best lifted onto a table or a well-padded locker. Really adequate control is, as a rule, best achieved by the following means. The child is made comfortable on the pillow or mattress and the back flexed as much as possible in order to separate the spinous processes of the vertebrae. The nurse then hooks one arm round the neck, the other round the crook of the flexed knees and allows her hands to meet in front of the patient, so forming a complete circle with her hands and arms and the child's

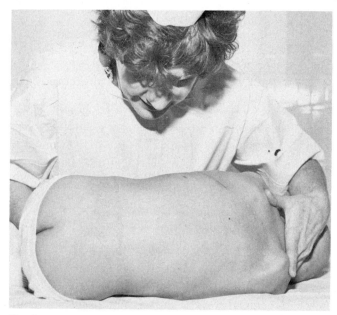

Fig. 40. Position for a lumbar puncture (a face mask may be worn by the nurse).

body (Fig. 40). Although safely restrained the child can breathe adequately and the nurse does not tire easily as the pull on her own hands gives her strength and support. The child should be adequately still, neither struggling nor crying while the pressure is being read, lest false readings be obtained.

Whenever it is thought that lumbar puncture may have to be done repeatedly, a sedative should be given so as to minimize possible fear and psychological trauma.

In children, headaches rarely follow lumbar puncture and the routine of keeping the patient flat and the foot of the bed raised is not necessary unless air has been injected as for the purpose of an air encephalogram.

Air encephalogram

The child should be prepared as for general anaesthesia. Under certain circumstances the procedure may be carried out under heavy sedation, but most commonly a general anaesthetic is given. The procedure is usually carried out in the X-ray department.

A lumbar puncture is performed in the usual way and several millilitres of cerebrospinal fluid are withdrawn. The fluid is replaced by filtered air or pure oxygen, injected through a syringe attached to the lumbar puncture needle. This process is repeated several times. The amount exchanged in this way depends upon the age of the child.

When the child is sat up, the air rises within the cerebro-spinal canal, like an air bubble rising in water. If there is no abnormality present, the ventricles of the brain will fill with air and their outline and position can be clearly seen on a radiograph. Air encephalogram is never carried out in cases of suspected space occupying lesions as these cause raised intracranial pressure and the withdrawal of cerebrospinal fluid may lead to 'coning' of the brain-stem through the foramen magnum into the spinal canal, resulting in sudden death from pressure on this vital part of the nervous system.

Ventriculography

For ventriculography the head has to be shaved, as the blunt cannula is introduced through the scalp, directly into the ventricles. In young infants this can be done through the still-open fontanelle or the still-ununited sutures. In older patients it is necessary to make burr holes in the skull. Approximately 40 ml of filtered air or pure oxygen is then injected after withdrawing a similar quantity of cerebrospinal fluid.

In either case, radiographs are taken immediately after the air has been injected. By placing the patient in different positions the movement of the air through the ventricular system and the shape, size and position of the ventricles can be clearly seen. Alternatively a filling defect of any part of the cerebrospinal or ventricular system will be a valuable aid to diagnosis. Ventriculography is used when a brain abscess or intracranial tumour is suspected.

Aftercare

1. Record temperature, pulse, respiration and blood pressure at frequent and regular intervals until stabilized.

2. Observe for signs of raised intracranial pressure which include:

> Vomiting unrelated to meals and without previous warning.
> Headache, which is sometimes eased when the head is raised.
> A tense, bulging anterior fontanelle.*
> Distension of the scalp veins.*
> Separation of sutures.*
> Increase in the circumference of the head.*
> Papilloedema.
> Slowing of pulse rate.
> Convulsions.
> Meningeal cry.
> Head retraction.
> Arching of the back.
> Internal strabismus.
> Irritability.
> Resentment at being touched.
> Drowsiness.

3. Keep the child quiet and comfortable. Give analgesics as prescribed for any headache.

---

* Applies to infants only.

Radio-opaque methods

Angiography is used when it is desirable to outline blood vessels of the brain. An injection of a radio-opaque dye is made into the main carotid artery in the neck. As the dye circulates through the arteries their outline can be seen on the X-ray screen or film. Pictures are taken in rapid succession. In this way abnormalities such as angiomata of the brain can be clearly seen and accurately located. Angiography is a valuable diagnostic aid, particularly prior to certain operations on the brain.

In cases of suspected non-communicating hydrocephalus, contrast or radio-opaque media may be injected into the ventricle through the anterior fontanelle or through burr holes, and the site of a hold-up may be seen in the radiograph. Radio-opaque substances may also be injected into the spinal cord to discover the site of a spinal tumour.

Possible complications

These may include: bleeding from injection site, hemiparesis, disturbances of blood pressure, convulsions, and infection.

Aftercare

1. Frequent observations of the injection site for any oozing or haematoma formation.

2. Pulse, temperature, respiration and blood pressure recordings at regular intervals.

3. Report any indication of speech disturbance, alteration in responsiveness or muscle weakness.

Electroencephalogram

It is known that rhythmical electric charges of a certain pattern and frequency are exhibited in the human brain and that both pattern and frequency change in disease. Recordings can be made by means of electrical leads placed on the patient's scalp. The graphs obtained are typical of certain diseases or abnormalities such as cerebral abscess or degenerative diseases and are a valuable aid to diagnosis. It is desirable to have a fully cooperative patient, capable of obeying instructions (e.g. to open or close his eyes) and this is often achieved by arranging for the mother or for the child's own nurse to be present. Frequently, however, a sedative has to be given.

Brain scan

This is a non-invasive technique which demonstrates any tumour or other pathology in the brain.

A radio-opaque substance is first given to the child either orally or intravenously. This radio-activity diffuses into any abnormal cerebral tissue and is picked up by the scanner which prints out the uptake as a picture.

It should be explained to the child before the procedure that he will need to lie quietly and still whilst it takes place.

EPILEPSY AND CONVULSIONS

'Epilepsy and convulsion should, like cough be regarded as symptoms rather than diagnostic entities'.

Brett, *'Children in Health and Disease'*

Febrile convulsions

These occur in about 5% of children under the age of 5 years, especially in those with a similar history in siblings or in a parent. The convulsion is associated with the rapid rise in temperature which may herald the onset of an infection. Immediate treatment is to control the convulsion with intravenous diazepam or clonazepam. The parents should also be given advice on how to prevent the convulsions from recurring: by giving aspirin orally and to keep the child cool whenever he becomes feverish. Some of these children may develop epilepsy later in life.

Infantile spasms

These usually begin between the age of 3–18 months. A typical attack involves repeated flexion of the head and trunk forward whilst the arms are raised up. Numerous attacks occur daily. The prognosis is poor. Commonly associated with mental handicap, the spasms may lead to major convulsions from about the age of 4 years.

Treatment is aimed at controlling the spasms with one of the anticonvulsants. Corticosteroids and ACTH have been used successfully in improving the associated EEG abnormality and also in reducing the number of attacks.

Petit mal

This rarely occurs before the age of 3 years.

Attacks of minor epilepsy may be so mild that they are only noticed by those who are in constant contact with the patient. The loss of consciousness is so fleeting that, after a momentary pause, the patient immediately resumes his activities as if nothing had happened. The eyes may take on a momentary dazed look or there may be a feeling of giddiness or a loss of postural control.

Major epilepsy

The stages of a major epileptic attack are the same in children as in adults, but children frequently become irritable or cling to their mothers as if seeking comfort during the period of aura. Occasionally there is no loss of consciousness nor are there true convulsive movements but the child shows considerable behaviour disturbances or temporary loss of memory and, in some cases, unexplained headaches or abdominal pain are thought to be of epileptic origin.

A variety of drugs are used to control convulsions. These include phenobarbitone, Mysolin, Epanutin or various combinations of anticonvulsant drugs. Some of these drugs have serious side-effects and the nurse should be well-informed about them, and make careful observations.

In dealing with a child in a convulsion, the principal concern is to keep him from harming himself. If he has been up and about the nurse should lay him on a bed or on the floor away from any harmful object. The child's head should be turned to the side to allow saliva to drain freely and so prevent inhalation. Tight clothing should be loosened. If the attack occurs in bed, pillows are best removed. Avoid restraint. If possible place a padded tongue blade between teeth to prevent damage, but do not attempt to force open clenched teeth.

As the patient regains consciousness he is likely to be bewildered, and reassurance and comfort should be given. A warm drink may help to send him into a restful sleep.

In hospital, a tray containing recovery instruments and swabs is usually kept near the beds of known epileptic children but this should be covered and out of sight of both child and visitors. While looking after the patient the nurse should make careful observations.

Observations

How did the fit start? Was there an aura, noise in the ears, or flash of light? Were there any movements? Where did they begin? Where did they spread to? Were the movements tonic or clonic? Was there a tremor and eye movements?

Did the patient lose consciousness? Were the eyes open or closed? If closed, could they be opened? Towards which side were they turned? If lightly touched, did the eyes blink? Was there incontinence, cyanosis, and/or breath holding? Did the patient bite his tongue? What was the duration of the fit? Was the patient drowsy after the fit or was he confused? Did the patient show abnormal or unusual behaviour after the fit? What could the patient remember about the fit?

General nursing management

The aim should always be that the child with epilepsy is encouraged to lead as normal a life as possible. Both the parents and the child should be given every opportunity to ask questions and to discuss freely the nature of the illness and of the fits.

Some of these children may have an associated degree of mental handicap although many are of normal or of high intelligence. Schooling provision should be considered on an individual basis in full consultation with the parents and the Education Authorities.

Behavioural disturbances, e.g. temper tantrums or over-activity, are common and psychiatric help may be indicated. Every encouragement and support should be given to the child to promote independence, e.g. in accepting responsibility for his own medication. The only limitations on physical activities should be that the child should not be allowed to swim or to climb on his own.

MENINGITIS (INFLAMMATION OF THE MENINGES)

Meningitis is more common in children than in adults. The main types are classified according to the causative organism:

1. Pyogenic, e.g. meningococci, pneumococci, staphylococci.
2. Viral or aseptic meningitis.
3. Tuberculous meningitis.

Presentation

Initial presentation depends upon the age of onset, but includes:

Headaches and pain in back of neck.

Vomiting and nausea.

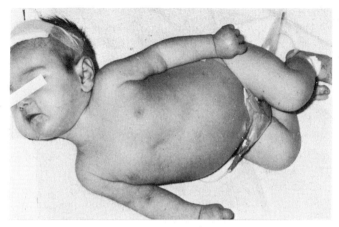

Fig. 41. Extreme opisthotonos due to cerebral irritation in a young baby.

    Fever.
    Irritability, restlessness with a high-pitched meningeal
      cry.
    Photophobia.
  Later signs:
    Increasing drowsiness.
    Resentful at being touched.
    Opisthotonos.
    Convulsions.

Diagnosis

    Established by lumbar puncture and laboratory examination of the cerebrospinal fluid. Blood culture and throat swabs should be taken, together with blood for a full blood count and electrolyte estimation.

Treatment

    Appropriate antibiotics either intramuscularly, intravenously or intrathecally.

Nursing management

1. Provide minimal nursing intervention in a quiet room or space that is compatible with the child's condition. Barrier nursing may be required to prevent the spread of infection (see p. 28).

2. Frequent observations to monitor child's response to treatment:

> Temperature, pulse and respiration.
> Blood pressure.
> Head circumference in the young infant should be measured.
> Neurological status and behaviour.
> Intake and output, to assess renal function.

3. Basic comfort care, particularly of pressure areas and mouth. Position semi-conscious or unconscious child on side and turn at regular intervals. Frequent suction to nasopharynx to prevent aspiration of secretions.

4. Assess nutritional status:

> Oral feeding if child is conscious and able to tolerate adequate amounts.
> Nasogastric feeding if child is semi-comatosed or unconscious.
> Intravenous infusion if dehydration is present and long-term feeding required.

Whatever route is chosen, the aim should be to provide at least sufficient kilojoules (Calories) to meet energy requirements and enough fluids to maintain hydration.

5. Provide stimulation as the child progresses with suitable play activities according to age and interests (see pp. 6–18).

6. Support for parents. Encourage their participation in care. Provide opportunities for questions to be asked about their child's progress and future.

Prognosis

In most instances complete recovery may be expected,

but much depends on early diagnosis and prompt, effective treatment. The outlook in most serious in very young infants and the prognosis should always be somewhat guarded.

Complications

Complications include neurological disturbances, hydro-cephalus, mental deficiency, paralysis, deafness and con-vulsions. A special point worth remembering is that, in young infants, meningitis may occur in a *sub-acute form*. There may be little or no fever; diarrhoea and vomiting may lead to dehydration and sunken eyes and fontanelle. Together with these misleading symptoms neurological ex-amination is difficult and often atypical in babies, and only lumbar puncture can confirm the diagnosis of meningitis.

ACUTE ENCEPHALITIS

Acute encephalitis may be caused by viral infections, specific fevers and, rarely, by vaccination.

Signs and symptoms

The onset of the disease is very acute with high fever, severe headache, vomiting, visual disturbances and some-times convulsions and loss of consciousness. Patients may be so confused as to become irrational and violent to an extent which necessitates restraint.

Treatment

Antibiotics may be given to treat any secondary infec-tion. Steroids are often prescribed although their value in the treatment of encephalitis is not clear.

Nursing management

Generally supportive and along the same lines as the care of a child with meningitis (see p. 286).

Tracheostomy and/or mechanical ventilation may be required for the comatosed child.

The prognosis is variable, emotional and behavioural problems are common in the convalescent phase of the illness which may be prolonged.

INTRACRANIAL TUMOUR

Intracranial, space-occupying lesions are fairly common, particularly in children of 5–10 years old. Treatment is surgical or by radiotherapy. According to their situation the lesions cause complications by pressure, e.g. pressure on the pituitary gland, causing diabetes insipidus. Some of these tumours are malignant and inoperable but in many cases there is reasonable hope of successful treatment. The commonest site is the cerebellum and the pressure here causes the patient to suffer from vomiting which is difficult to control. Papilloedema is usually present and the child is grossly ataxic.

Nursing management

Care will need to be related to the individual child's treatment and general condition. The aims will include the alleviation of pain and other distressing symptoms, and the provision of emotional support to the parents and child.

CEREBRAL PALSY

Cerebral palsy is caused by defect or disease of the brain affecting the upper motor neurones and is liable to occur any time before, during or after birth. The disease is not progressive.

Children suffering from cerebral palsy have difficulty in

carrying out coordinated movements. The adductor muscles of the thigh in particular go into spasm (the scissor attitude). The gait is unsteady or clumsy, and is often reminiscent of a drunken man, charging forward, dragging a foot and stumbling about, or the movements may be slow and writhing. The incoordination of the respiratory muscles leads to frequent chest infections. Speech is difficult if the lip, tongue and laryngeal muscles are affected and the child may grimace in an attempt at forming words. What speech is possible is often explosive and the abnormal functioning of the respiratory muscles causes the child to make uncontrolled, animal-like noises. This may intensify the impression that the child is mentally abnormal. In addition he has difficulty in swallowing and he may have a constant dribble of saliva down his chin. Poor mastication causes dental decay, anaemia and malnutrition.

Many spastic children have a squint caused by muscle spasm, and visual disturbances such as double vision are common. Hearing defects are often associated with cerebral palsy, and these and the visual defects are often partly responsible for the delay in acquiring speech and learning to read.

Nursing management and treatment

The aim is to make a full assessment and then set to work on those muscle groups and abilities which give hope of response and seem capable of development. Teamwork is the essence in the treatment of cerebral palsy.

This 'teamwork' concept will need to include the parents and other members of the child's family as participants in order to be fully effective.

The education of the child with cerebral palsy must depend to some extent on the degree of handicap. The new technology of electronics and silicone chips has made enormous advances in developing aids to help these children, even for those with severe motor problems.

SPINA BIFIDA

Spina bifida is a congenital abnormality due to a defect in the formation of the skeletal arch enclosing the spinal cord. It occurs most frequently in the lumbar region but may be present anywhere along the spinal column or even on the skull.

There are various degrees of this abnormality. In the mildest there is nothing beyond the bony defect. At other times a patch of hair or naevus over the spinal defect should lead the nurse to suspect the presence of spina bifida. Next in severity is the meningocele, in which case the spinal meninges herniate and the sac contains cerebrospinal fluid. If the sac contains nerve tissue as well as fluid the lesion is called meningomyelocele.

When a baby with a spina bifida is born, immediate steps should be taken to assess the problem and prepare for possible surgery, the lesion must be kept moist with saline soaks or with a bland non-adherent, non-greasy dressing such as Nusan B, as any damage at this stage may aggravate the neurological damage, already present. Paediatric surgeons generally feel that early surgery should be restricted to those with mild or moderate neurological involvement.

The operation, which should ideally take place within hours of birth, aims at giving the lesion a good cover of skin. The skin is undermined, often right round to the umbilicus, and drawn together over the meningocele. Direct suture is usually possible after the underlying sac of meninges has been excised. The skin cover gives good protection, prevents infection (e.g. meningitis), helps to reduce paralysis and makes the care of the baby easier for all concerned.

Post-operative management and care

1. Maintenance of a clear airway together with careful positioning of the infant to protect the operative site and to relieve wound tension. The infant may be nursed prone or,

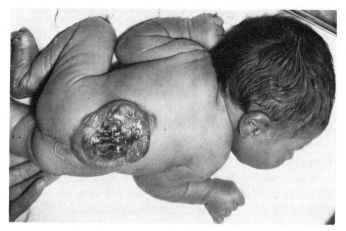

Fig. 42. A newborn infant with meningomyelocele.

alternatively, in slings suspended from the roof of the
incubator.

2. Nutrition. Oral feeding can usually be commenced
4–6 hours post-operatively depending upon the infant's
condition. A nasogastric tube may be kept in position for a
few hours after operation for aspiration of stomach contents at frequent intervals.

3. Prevention of infection:

 Daily dressings only when indicated by the surgeon.

 Application of urine bag or tube to prevent soiling of
  the dressing.

 Monitor body temperature.

4. Measure and chart head circumference daily to detect
developing hydrocephalus. Early signs of developing
hydrocephalus include a tense fontanelle.

5. Wound care. Suction drains usually removed about 48
hours after operation, sutures about 8–10 days later.

6. Family support. Encourage parents to visit and handle
their baby. Talk over their baby's progress with them and

answer all questions. Be prepared for a repetition of questions which is a result of natural anxiety (see p. 72).

7. Physiotherapy. Passive exercises will need to be provided initially by physiotherapists and later the parents should be instructed in how to continue with the programme at home.

8. Prepare parents for discharge. Liaise with the paediatric liaison health visitor to ensure continuity of care.

Conservative care

When surgery is delayed or even impossible, nurses should then use their ingenuity in the way they protect the protruding lesion. Polyurethane rings are most satisfactory.

Special care should be taken to prevent trophic ulceration and to keep these babies warm, bearing in mind the fact that many are paralysed and lack sensory appreciation.

Feeds often need to be small and frequent, taking account of fluid and calorie requirements.

Long-term care

The degree of handicap varies from one child to another, and each poses a different set of problems. Whilst each must be considered individually, the main areas of concern can be considered under the following headings.

Urinary problems may range from stress incontinence to complete loss of sphincter control. Some children develop over-distending bladders with the consequent risk of infection which will require intensive treatment with antibiotics. Where the bladder becomes over-distended, a method of manual expression of urine can be taught to the mother and later the child. Girls, particularly, present difficult problems; if incontinence pads and protective plastic pants do not provide the answer a urinary diversion may become necessary. The usual technique is to divert the ureters into an isolated segment of the ileum, of which one end is closed and the other brought out on to the anterior abdominal wall. A disposable bag can then be fitted to collect the urine. Boys can use a penile clamp or a fitted penile urinal. It is important to ensure that these children can take plenty of fluids by mouth.

Bowel control. Most of these children can achieve bowel continence with good management. This involves giving a low residue diet together with an enema once or twice a week.

Voluntary defecation can also be achieved in some children, by straining at stool after a meal or hot drink. Care must be taken that the rectum does not become impacted with faeces thus causing overflow incontinence.

Orthopaedic handicaps. Intensive physiotherapy, training and splinting will all help in the management of any limb deformities. Most of these children can be taught to walk using calipers although great care must be taken in view of the skin anaesthesia which makes them very vulnerable to trophic sores and ulceration. Some children will need to use a wheelchair and a surprising agility can often be achieved, sometimes to the envy of their friends!

Hydrocephalus. Although hydrocephalus will usually have been treated with the insertion of a shunt system, the treatment itself may lead to difficulties and complications. The tubes may need to be lengthened as the child grows or the shunt may become blocked and needs to be replaced urgently. Occasionally, the tubes themselves may become disconnected, and need surgical correction. Low grade, persistent septicaemia, most commonly due to *Staphylococcus albus* may occur and this is difficult to control until the valve is removed.

Social and psychological problems. Children with physical handicaps are not necessarily also emotionally disturbed, but research findings do suggest that these children tend to be less mature and more disturbed than those without any handicap. Mental handicap too may present a problem, although the intelligence level varies and is usually related to the type of defect.

HYDROCEPHALUS

Hydrocephalus is the name given to an excessive accumulation of cerebrospinal fluid within the skull. The resulting pressure causes the skull bones to separate, the skull circumference to increase, the ventricles to become distended and the substance of the brain to be compressed.

The excess accumulation is produced by obstruction of the flow or absorption of the fluid, due to congenital malformation, birth injury, inflammatory processes or pressure from a tumour.

In the *communicating type* there is a block within the subarachnoid space although there is free communication between the ventricular system and the spinal theca.

In the *non-communicating type*, the outflow from within the brain to the subarachnoid space is blocked.

In some cases the abnormality is slight and may arrest spontaneously.

Presentation

1. Increased intracranial pressure from obstruction of cerebrospinal fluid circulation leads to separation of the skull sutures and increasing skull circumference measurement.

2. The skull appears abnormal in shape and size, with a bulging brow which often seems to dwarf the face.

3. The fontanelles are tense and palpate.

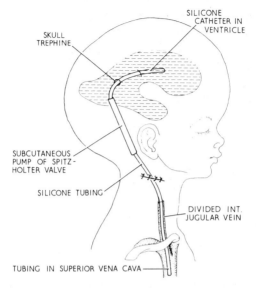

Fig. 43. Diagram of a child with hydrocephalus treated with the aid of a Spitz-Holter valve.

4. The eyes show a downward deviation—the 'setting sun' sign, as the white of the sclera is visible above the iris.

5. Vomiting, failure to thrive and irritability, together with delayed development, are often noticed very early on in the condition.

Treatment and nursing management

After confirmation of hydrocephalus by radiography and other special investigations (see p. 280), surgical treatment may be indicated. By means of a fine tube and a one-way valve, e.g. Spitz-Holter, the cerebrospinal fluid is diverted from the ventricles into the blood stream or other body cavity, e.g. the atria of the heart.

Pre-operative care

If the child has been vomiting for some time, nutrition and hydration may be a problem. Offer small but frequent feeds with extra clear fluids.

In view of the raised intracranial pressure, minimum nursing care disturbance to avoid increasing irritability. Plan for care of pressure areas, eye care to be completed before feeding whenever possible.

Encourage parents to participate in care as much as possible. Provide facilities for parents to be resident if they wish to be. Answer all their questions about the care being provided, and explain the need for investigations and surgery. If the child is old enough explain all the treatments, etc. in a language he can understand.

Prepare for surgery as for any other operation that involves the use of general anaesthesia.

Shaving the child's head. In order to avoid undue distress for the child, the head is shaved in the anaesthetic room after the anaesthetic has been administered. The hair should be shampooed the day before operation and any scalp infection should be treated.

Post-operative care

Nursing action	Explanation
Frequent observations of pulse, respiration, temperature, blood pressure and neurological status.	Initially to detect signs of haemorrhage, shock and increased intracranial pressure. Later to indicate infection or blocked valve.
Change position of child every two hours.	To prevent pressure areas becoming sore.
Head of child should be raised.	To promote drainage of cerebrospinal fluid through shunt.

Nursing action	Explanation
Avoid positioning of child on site of valve until wound is well healed.	To avoid damaging the overlying skin.
Nasogastric tube may be in situ on free drainage particularly if a rentriculoperitoneal shunt is performed.	To avoid abdominal distension.
Commence feeding gradually, 4–6 hours post-operatively. Administer intravenous fluids as prescribed. Measure and record fluid intake and output.	To maintain hydration and nutrition. Provide oral pleasure and comfort.
Frequent mouth and eye care.	To prevent dryness of mucous membranes and avoid infection.
Pump or 'milk' valve only as directed by surgeon.	To promote drainage where indicated.
As child progresses plan play activities appropriate to interests and development.	To prevent mental stimulation.
Involve parents in care, giving explanation where necessary.	Preparation for discharge home.
Parents should be taught to detect complications and seek medical advice for fever, dehydration, redness/swelling of operation site and headache/irritability.	Infection. Shunt malfunction.

SOME BEHAVIOUR PROBLEMS

Enuresis

A child who repeatedly passes urine involuntarily at an age when he can normally be expected to be toilet-trained is said to be suffering from enuresis. He may either never have been dry, or may have relapsed after a period of normal control of micturition. Wetting may occur several times a night, very occasionally, or perhaps once or twice per month.

Causes include renal infections, nephrosis, diabetes, psychological disturbances, congenital abnormalities of the urinary tract, spina bifida, neurological lesions, mental handicap, chronic constipation, and intestinal worms. A frequent cause is behaviour disturbance following the birth of a new baby, a change to a new school, a severe illness or other experience causing a loss of security.

A thorough physical examination, urinalysis and full investigations of the renal tract must be done to exclude organic disease, and if these are negative, psychological treatment may be advised. This will include full enquiry into home background, and the parents will be interviewed as well as the child. They may be advised to restrict fluid intake during the evening, to rouse the child and offer a pot before they themselves go to bed and to leave a small light burning. Punishment and scolding are, as a rule, out of place, although an overworked exasperated mother may well be forgiven if she loses patience with the child. Constant wet sheets may be a great trial in a small town flat and criticism from neighbours is not easy to bear.

Every small improvement should be hailed as a hopeful sign and encouragement and praise given whenever possible. Sometimes drugs are used such as the tricyclic anti-depressants. A 'conditioned reflex' can be created in older children by using a specially designed buzzer which goes off and rouses the child as he starts to void urine. Properly used these may score successes in 75% of cases treated.

Faecal incontinence (encopresis)

Faecal incontinence, i.e. soiling at an age when a child may reasonably be expected to be toilet-trained, may be due to a number of reasons. A common cause is constipation with overflow, and reasons for this situation range from 'pot refusal' due to painful anal fissure in toddlers, to emotional disturbances, congenital abnormalities and bad housing conditions. Another example is the child who notes his mother's distress if he does not have his bowels open regularly and uses bowel function to attract attention, 'please' or 'punish'. Sometimes the lavatory itself is to blame: it may be situated on a dark landing in an old tenement building or in the garden, or it may be so high that the child dreads using it for fear of falling in.

The cause of faecal incontinence should therefore be investigated very carefully and patiently. Good teamwork between parents, paediatrician, child guidance clinic and health visitor will usually cure the condition.

MENTAL HANDICAP

Mental handicap or mental defect can be defined as inadequate mental development resulting in incapacity for independent social and intellectual adaptation in everyday life. There are many causes for this handicap which can be classified into the following groups:

(1) Genetically determined, e.g. Down's syndrome.
(2) Antenatal infection, e.g. rubella or syphilis.
(3) Birth injury.
(4) Postnatal, e.g. encephalitis, cerebral infection, trauma.

Mental handicap may also be associated with other handicaps, e.g. cerebral palsy or the child with hydro-cephalus and myelomeningocele.

Only a few types of mental handicap are obvious at birth, such as Down's syndrome or microcephaly, whilst with others the condition may be unsuspected for several months. The first indication of this handicap in the young child is usually noticed in a delay by the child to reach the normal milestones in sitting, standing and walking; speech too is delayed. The child often appears placid and 'good' or conversely may appear hyperactive, restless and difficult to feed. Occasionally the handicap is only recognized when the child starts school and has difficulty in learning the three 'Rs'.

Whatever the cause and whenever it is diagnosed the news will cause much anxiety and distress for the parents and the family. The parents may vacillate between extreme feelings of total rejection of their child to overwhelming possessiveness which may lead to neglect of their older children. The parents often try to find a cause for the handicap and may blame themselves. The nurse must recognize that these feelings are very real to the parents who will need much support and help in adopting a positive acceptance of their child's handicap. Many parents benefit from having contact with parents in a similar situation and help, both practical and emotional, is provided by voluntary agencies for the handicapped child.

The parents will have many questions to ask, wanting to know what their child's potential will be, how best to help him and what type of schooling will be needed? In order to answer these questions a complete assessment will be made by the multidisciplinary team concerned with the care for the child. Measurements of the intelligence quotient will be made by the clinical psychologist and compared with the chronological age; physical ability will be assessed by the physiotherapist, social behaviour by the nurse and the child's medical history thoroughly investigated by the paediatrician. Even with this initial assessment it is difficult to forecast how the child will develop and progress. Assessment therefore should be carried out periodically in order that appropriate stimulation and training is given at the right stage of development.

Parents will need to know that their mentally handicapped child requires more and not less of the normal childhood pleasures and activities. It is through play, nursery rhymes, songs and stories that the young child learns. He should be cuddled, praised and made a fuss of so that he feels secure and will want to do his best. As far as possible the parents should treat the child normally whilst recognizing that because of this handicap he will be slower and less able than other children of the same age.

All children whatever their disability are able to go to school. Special schooling with small groups of children and specially qualified teachers provide education and training that is geared to the individual child's needs and potential.

In the past many mentally handicapped children were placed in large institutions for care and protection where they were often forgotten by their families. It is now recognized that with training and care many more mentally handicapped people can take their place in society where they may work in sheltered workshops and live in a hostel if there is no family home.

However it is important to recognize that many children because of their handicap or social background may require admission into a specialist hospital; here doctors and nurses with special expertise will provide an environment which will give the child the opportunity to learn social skills and to be cared for. Even though care must be planned in the long term, parents are encouraged to maintain family links joining in hospital and ward activities and where possible taking their child home for weekends and holidays.

As with all children the mentally handicapped child may need admission into the paediatric unit with a superimposed medical or surgical condition. The nurse should especially remember how distressing this situation will be for the child. In order to avoid too much bewilderment and distress the child should, whenever possible, be looked after by 'his nurse'. Every effort should be made to follow the child's home routine whilst he is in hospital in order to maintain the progress he is making. Facilities for mother or father to be resident should be provided.

Further reading

CUNNINGHAM, C. (1982) *Down's Syndrome*. London: Souvenir Press.

DRILLIEN, C. M. & DRUMMAND, M. B. (1977) *Neurodevelopmental Problems in Early Childhood*. Oxford: Blackwell Scientific.

HOPKINS, A. (1981) *Epilepsy*. Oxford: Oxford University Press.

HOSKING, G. (1982) *An Introduction to Paediatric Neurology*. London: Faber & Faber.

ISAACSON, R. (1974) *The Retarded Child*. Illinois: Argus Communications.

JENNETT, B. (1977) *An Introduction to Neurosurgery*, 3rd edn. London: Heinemann Medical.

TILL, K.(1975) *Paediatric Neurosurgery*. London: Blackwell Scientific.

13 Disorders involving the skin

INFANTILE ECZEMA

Infantile eczema is an allergic skin condition seen in varying degrees of severity. In mild cases only the flexor surfaces of the legs and arms are affected, in severe cases the rash may cover most of the body including the cheeks, forehead and scalp.

Infantile eczema mostly affects very young children. It is rarely seen before the age of 3 months and with the exception of localized patches may be expected to clear up by the age of 2–3 years. A definite family history of eczema, asthma or hay fever is typical and some children who suffer from eczema in infancy develop asthma later in life.

Boys are more frequently affected than girls and the babies are often blue-eyed, fair-haired and frequently delightful patients to look after. Allergy to certain foods such as eggs, fish, cow's milk and certain pollen or household dust can sometimes be found, either by taking a careful history or by performing intradermal tests.

Signs and symptoms

The rash is commonly first noticed over the forehead, cheeks and scalp but the areas around the mouth stay clear. As the eczema spreads the flexures of the elbows and knees and the folds behind the ears become affected and patchy areas may occur in any part of the body. Initially the skin is red, hot and scaly but soon papules and vesicles appear and as they break down clear serum exudes from the lesion.

This is known as weeping eczema and at this stage the skin easily becomes infected. Irritation is intense and it may be almost impossible to stop the infant from scratching. As the exudate dries up thick crusts are formed. In spite of the extensive lesions, eczema leaves no scars.

Treatment

Treatment often includes a full investigation of the possible exciting causes. Intradermal tests with specific proteins, pollen or dust may show a positive reaction to a certain agent which can then be eliminated from the diet or the child's environment. Psychological disturbances may be present and both parents and patient need guidance and psychotherapy.

Local treatment and nursing management

This includes the use of coal tar preparations, calamine lotion with or without an oily base and the addition of a mild antiseptic. Ointment containing hydrocortisone may be ordered for local application. This should be applied with care remembering that absorption of cortisone can lead to dangerous complications. Unguent emulsifications may be added to bath water or alternatively applied to lesions. This preparation whilst replacing soap allays irritation, is soothing and assists with the separation of crusts. The child usually enjoys the bath, giving mother an opportunity to make a special fuss of her child. A soft towel should be used for drying. The skin is gently dabbed and never rubbed as this is abrasive to healing skin.

The local applications vary according to the stage of the rash. When dry and scaly, creams are usually ordered. They are either applied direct to the skin and left exposed, or spread thinly onto gauze and bandaged in place with an open-weave bandage. Tubular gauze is also useful for keeping a dressing comfortably in place. Infected areas may be treated with antiseptic lotion.

General nursing management

Nursing action

Keep the child cool. Clothing should be light and made of cotton. Alternatively may be left without any clothing on. Ambient temperature should be 70°F to avoid hypothermia.

Nails kept clean and short.

Occupation. Suitable play activities and education as appropriate should be provided according to the individual child's needs.

Parental participation. Every effort should be made to support and encourage the involvement of parents in care. Facilities for the mother or father to be resident should be provided.

Restraint to limbs using tubular gauze. This should be avoided whenever possible, but if necessary should be applied by a qualified nurse and released at regular intervals.

Diet. A nursing/medical history will indicate any allergy to specific foods, e.g. eggs or cow's milk.

Sedatives. Antihistamines may be prescribed.

Explanation

Will help to relieve irritation and incidence of scratching.

To prevent secondary infection.

Will help to divert the child's attention from the skin irritation whilst helping to meet normal developmental needs.

Important to the child's normal emotional developmental needs. Will help to allay anxiety and frustration, thus reducing the likelihood of further scratching and will help to promote healing.

Scratching of the skin produces further damage to the epithelial cells and increases the risk of introducing infection.

Eliminate those items from the diet to help reduce extent of the eczema.

Will reduce irritation.

Immunization and vaccination

Children with eczema can be treated as any others with regard to immunization programmes in the British Isles.

ACNE VULGARIS

This very common and distressing condition occurs at puberty. It is due to an excessive output and overgrowth of sebaceous glands particularly on the face, chest and shoulders. Blockage of sebum occurs and a comedo or 'black head' is produced.

Treatment

It is of utmost importance to reduce the greasiness of the skin. The face should be washed in hot water as often as possible and the comedos removed with a comedo extractor. Calamine lotion with 3% sulphur is then applied and rubbed in well. Topical peroxide preparations or vitamin A acid have in some instances been helpful.

Long-term tetracycline therapy has been found to be of value in severe cases. The patient is always very self-conscious about these spots and will need constant reassurance that once puberty is over these lesions will disappear, but that squeezing of the spots produces scars and should be avoided.

General preventative guidance

Wash the face gently at least twice daily.

Shampoo hair daily or as frequently as possible.

Continue the above regime even after the face clears.

Diet does not appear to make any difference, but occasionally a patient may feel that a certain food worsens the condition, e.g. chocolate, which is then best avoided.

IMPETIGO CONTAGIOSA

Impetigo is a skin infection caused by the streptococcus or staphylococcus. It is very common in children of school age and spreads easily, particularly in overcrowded homes with

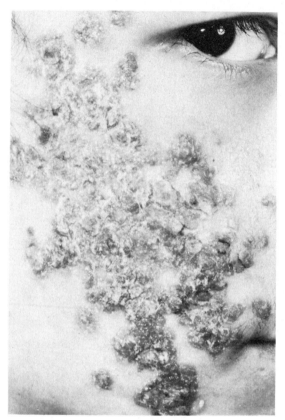

Fig. 44. A typical case of severe impetigo.

poor hygiene. The organism enters the skin through a crack or a scratch and for that reason is often associated with an infested head.

At first small vesicles appear and as they break the lesion becomes red and weeping and as the exudate dries up thick crusts form. Typical sites are on the scalp, the chin and around the lips. The crusts have the appearance of being 'stuck on'.

Local treatment

Local treatment consists in softening the crusts with warm saline bathings or a solution of potassium permanganate 1 : 4000. The skin may be painted with an antiseptic preparation such as boracic cream or an antibiotic cream. Occasionally antibiotics may be ordered by mouth if the infection is severe or fails to respond to local treatment.

The child suffering from impetigo is likely to infect others and if admitted to hospital should be nursed with barrier precautions. Crockery and cutlery should be sterilized until the last lesion has healed. Scratching is prevented in the same way, as in the case of infantile eczema (see p. 305).

The condition may clear within a few days and rarely leaves any scars. Recurrence should be prevented by giving the mother guidance with regard to personal hygiene and building up the child's general resistance, by good diet, exercise in the fresh air and an adequate vitamin intake.

N.B. If the child is being cared for at home he should be kept away from his school or playgroup until the lesions have healed. Inform the health visitor or school nurse when the diagnosis has been made.

BURNS AND SCALDS

Burns and scalds are among the most frequently occurring accidents in childhood (some thousand patients are admitted annually to hospitals in the London area alone) and they are the more tragic, because so many of them are preventable.

Common causes of burns and scalds in children

1. Open fires left unprotected.
2. Mirrors, pictures and attractive ornaments placed above electric fires or open fires attract children to reach for them.

3. Saucepans containing hot fluids with their handles left jutting out on stoves within the reach of children.

4. Tablecloths which can be pulled by a young child so that the items on the table fall over, including teapots, cups, etc. containing very hot fluids.

5. Baths filled with hot water before cold so that the young child is scalded on buttocks or feet on immersion into the bath.

6. Playing with matches.

7. Playing with fireworks.

Prevention

1. A fire should always be guarded when young children are about.

2. Advise parents to remove items from above a fireplace.

3. Always invert saucepan handles on any stove.

4. With young children in a family tablecloths should not be used. The table may be protected either with place mats or with a short plastic non-slip cover.

5. Always fill a bath with at least 1 inch of cold water before running in the hot.

6. Never allow children to handle matches until old enough to be instructed in their proper use.

7. Firework parties should always be supervised and managed by responsible adults. Children should never have free access to loose fireworks.

Classification of burns and scalds

Modern surgery refers to only two degrees of burns and scalds: superficial burns, and full thickness or deep burns. As a rule *superficial burns* may be expected to heal with little scarring, while *full thickness* burns are slow to heal and may cause scarring, crippling contractions and loss of function, and usually require skin grafting and prolonged and repeated treatment in hospital.

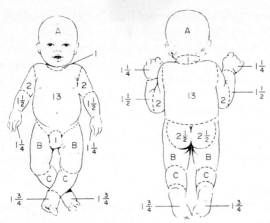

Fig. 45. The Lund and Browder method of measuring burns (from Lund, C. C. & Browder, N. N., *Surg. Gynec. Obstet.*).

The extent of the burn is as important as the depth. For purposes of classification the 'Waller Method' is frequently used. The body surface is divided into sections of 9% of the total and thus, with reference to a chart, it is easy to estimate the extent of the burn as being a multiple of 9%. The seriousness of the burn or scald is often far more dependent on the extent of the affected area, than on the thickness. A child may lose his life with an 18% superficial burn but an older patient may be expected to survive deep burns covering 50% of the body surface.

The Lund & Browder method of estimating the extent of burns is shown in Fig. 45. As in Waller's 'Rule of Nines' method, the body is divided into areas each of which is given a percentage value, but the values of certain areas alter with age as the proportions of the child's body are changed by normal growth.

Treatment for shock

No time should be lost in treating shock, even if the usual

Table 7. Table showing how the extent of a burn in certain areas of a child's body changes with age.

Areas affected by growth	Age				
	1 month	1 year	5 years	10 years	15 years
A = half of head	9½	8½	6½	5½	4½
B = half of one thigh	2¾	3¼	4	4¼	4½
C = half of one lower leg	2½	2½	2¾	3	3¼

symptoms may at first not be evident because shock is delayed. Shock is always directly proportionate to the area involved, as the loss of salts, protein and fluids into the tissue spaces and onto the body surface reduces the volume of circulating blood. The body reacts to this by a drop in blood pressure, subnormal temperature, pallor, thirst, restlessness and failure to secrete urine.

Intravenous therapy. This should be started immediately in all cases in which the area involved exceeds 9% of the body surface. It is usual to take blood for grouping and haemoglobin estimation before starting the infusion.

Plasma or the modern dextrans are the fluids of choice although fresh blood may be given according to the level of the haemoglobin which should never be allowed to fall below 70%.

The rate of fluid loss is estimated by repeated haematocrit readings, the haemoconcentration and the amount of urinary output. On the first day approximately two-thirds of the fluid loss is replaced in the first 8 hours after admission. After that, chemical tests of both blood and urine are done at least daily and the findings are taken as a guide for further intravenous therapy.

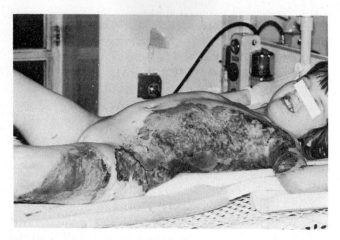

Fig. 46. Extensive burns. Child being nursed using the exposed method on foam pads which are changed frequently.

Oxygen therapy. Shock and the loss of red blood cells from the burnt surface may cause sufficient reduction in the oxygenating power of the blood to make oxygen therapy necessary. This is usually best given by mask as oxygen given by means of a tent interferes with local treatment and influences bacterial growth.

General nursing management

Admission. The child should be admitted to a cubicle, and barrier techniques used in order to protect the child from infection (see p. 28).

Swabs for laboratory culture should be taken from the burned areas. Sterile bed linen should be used. The child's weight should be recorded as the basis for calculating drug dosage and intravenous therapy.

At this stage the child should never be left alone. His

parents will need considerable support and reassurance during this time, especially as it is likely they will be suffering some shock themselves as a result of the accident.

Nursing observations. Observations of the child's appearance, pulse rate and blood pressure should be made frequently, as they are of considerable importance in assessing the child's general progress. In addition any girl with extensive burns (more than 10% surface area) should have an in-dwelling catheter in the bladder, and any boy should have Paul's tubing attached to the penis, so that urine output can be measured and recorded hourly. A rising pulse rate, hypotension and oliguria are all indications that the infusion rate should be increased to meet the body's fluid requirements. The nurse should realize that shivering and vomiting in these children are more likely to be due to inadequate fluid replacement or infection than to their being cold.

Diet. Oral fluids should be commenced as soon as possible after admission to the ward and are best given at this stage as 5% glucose 40 ml/kg/24 hours. It may be necessary to pass a nasogastric tube in order to avoid disturbing the child too much. Once the shock associated with the injury has passed, usually in about 2–3 days, the child should be given a diet high in protein and kilojoules. It may be necessary for this to be continued for several weeks, for much protein is lost from the burns and healing is delayed by malnutrition. Initially the child may be given a fortified milk preparation if necessary through a nasogastric tube.

Iron is necessary to combat anaemia. As soon as the patient can tolerate it, a full diet is given which is augmented by eggs, milk, vitamins and foods which are rich in iron. Such foods are red meat, liver, kidney, sardines, black treacle, wholemeal and rye bread and Bovril and Marmite.

As most of these foods are both palatable and colourful, there should be little difficulty in arranging attractive meals. The food intake must be measured accurately and the amounts taken should be known and supplemented by tube feeding if necessary. Much patience and ingenuity may be needed to achieve the necessary fluid and kilojoule intake.

Drug therapy. A broad spectrum antibiotic or a combination of one of these with penicillin is given prophylactically for the first 24 hours. The drug may then be changed according to the sensitivity report. Some surgeons change the drug routinely every time the patient has to be taken to the theatre, in order to guard against his becoming resistant to any one drug.

Morphine (0.05 mg/kg body weight) is a suitable sedative and analgesic to give to the child who will be frightened as well as in pain. This should always be relieved, as pain does exacerbate shock. The nurse should remember that this drug should not be given subcutaneously for the first day or so, as in the presence of shock it may not be adequately absorbed until later, with dangerous results. Initially the intravenous route is used.

Usually by 48 hours pain subsides and drugs such as codeine or phenobarbitone are sufficient. Elixir Phenergan has a sedative effect and at the same time reduces tissue swelling. It may have to be continued for some time and should never be withheld merely for fear of forming a habit.

Local treatment and nursing management

Treatment of the burnt area depends upon the extent of its surface and the part of the body involved. Prevention of infection, healing and early grafting, leading to early functioning of the part affected, are the desired goals.

Two methods may be used, the exposed or the closed method.

Exposure or open method. Children are often best nursed by the exposure method, which has the advantage of inhibiting bacterial growth by keeping the area cool, dry and exposed to light, and eliminating painful dressings while promoting healing with a minimum of scarring. The patient can move around freely and observation of the progress is possible; both these considerations are of psychological and clinical importance. Few dressings under anaesthetic are necessary and this means, among other things, that nutrition is not constantly being interrupted.

The affected area and surrounding skin are usually cleansed with a solution of 1% cetrimide or of Hibitane 1:2000. Large, heavy blisters may be punctured and drained but small ones are left and dead skin is not removed unless it is very dirty.

A hard, dry crust of plasma exudate usually forms within 24–36 hours and provides a sterile covering for the underlying surface. Air is allowed to circulate freely to aid the drying process and for that purpose special beds, polyurethane pads, extensions and slings may be used and the patient's position changed according to need. Using an aerosol spray, topical antibiotics can be applied, e.g. polymyxin and bacitracin. Pressure on the affected part must be avoided as a good blood supply is essential to healing.

Crusts begin to peel off after approximately 3 weeks when new epidermis has formed. Very thick crusts may be loosened by liquid paraffin soaks (gauze swabs saturated with paraffin) which are renewed every 4 hours. After approximately 12 hours, much of the crust can be lifted off with the aid of sterile forceps. This should only be done if the treatment is entirely painless, i.e. adequate healing underneath the crust has taken place.

Full thickness burns are treated in the same way initially, but after 1–2 weeks the patient is taken to the theatre for thorough examination and wound toilet. By now it is possible to decide how much of the tissue is dead and consequently incapable of primary healing. As a rule partial thickness burns may be expected to heal in 3–4 weeks, but full thickness burns will require grafting and are usually associated with some degree of deformity. Any sloughs are removed and skin grafting is undertaken. This operation is called *escharectomy* (eschar = slough). Loss of blood may be considerable but by now the patient's general condition should be so much better that he can stand up to operation even though further blood transfusion may be necessary.

In ideal conditions the grafted areas will be left exposed following operation.

Closed or dressed method. If the areas have been covered with dressings and bandages, it is important that the nurse should watch any exposed and pendant parts (the extremities particularly) for oedema and bleeding. Either must be reported at once. The bandaging requires great skill as considerable pressure is required in order to prevent blood or exudate from lifting the graft off its bed. At the same time it is obviously dangerous to apply the crêpe bandages too tightly. Oedema may be severe and may cause the bandage to become tight and impede circulation with consequent death of the skin graft. Nursing methods, such as elevating the part, are attempted to reduce the swelling before interfering with the bandage as this is often applied with the intention of correcting deformities and contractions, as well as covering the operation area.

Complications

Damage of liver and kidneys, pneumonia, reactions to blood transfusion, sepsis, uraemia and psychological disturbances are common. Treatment of any of these at the earliest stage is essential and in many cases these complications can be avoided by adequate medical and nursing care. Local complications may arise from sloughs and crusts which by their position or extent may restrict chest movement or the blood supply to extremities, causing chest complications or thrombosis and gangrene of the parts. Burns and scalds of the eyelids are likely to cause contractions followed by exposure of the cornea, resulting in keratitis. Careful swabbing may prevent complications but in some cases it is deemed best to temporarily stitch the upper and lower lid margins together or to excise the contracted lids and graft them.

Burns of the hands and external genitalia present further problems which have to be dealt with as the individual case demands. Warm baths will help the child to 'kick out' any contractures although splinting with Kramer wire or Plaster of Paris may still be necessary. The application of lanolin or Anthisan cream will help to soften healed areas and grafts.

Lesions of groins, neck and armpits should be prevented from contracting by separating them or extending them fully with the aid of pillows or rolls of polyurethane foam. Steam scalds of face, neck and tongue may require tracheostomy and so add to the already difficult nursing problem.

Emotional welfare

However exacting the routine nursing care, no nurse must ever forget the emotional welfare of these children. They are usually severely shocked and numbed in the first hours but after this initial stage they need a great deal of assurance, company and occupation. They are frightened by the accident and the sudden admission to hospital and often haunted by memories of the burst of flames and by feelings of guilt. Flame burns in particular, cause severe nightmares after 2 or 3 days, and the children easily develop feelings of resentment and a bad relationship towards their parents.

The presence of the mother for as much time as possible is of great psychological value. Any relatives or neighbours involved in the accident should be allowed to visit and speak to the child in order to reassure him. Sometimes it is possible to admit the mother with the child, provided she can spare the time from her other commitments. She can help to feed her child and play with him and sometimes may get him to sleep when he is wakeful or frightened. The idea that the mother can only be admitted or frequent visiting be arranged during the first days when the child is better, is completely mistaken. *It is in the first, initial stages that comfort from the mother is so important*. It is useless to cure a child physically while allowing psychological damage to persist or to develop.

Although a physiotherapist will carry out daily treatment to prevent and correct contractions and bad posture, mothers can often be taught to assist, e.g. when games are played to encourage deep breathing and so help to prevent chest infections. As soon as possible full occupation is needed to keep these patients happy.

Boredom encourages scratching and picking at the crusts, both of which may lead to infection, delayed healing and unnecessary scarring. Adequate occupation and company are far better means of preventing this than sedation or restraint. Toys and occupational material must at first be of the sterilizable kind. In situations of stress such as this, the child should not be deprived of a loved toy and if this cannot be sterilized even a teddy bear can be covered by a clean polythene bag.

It is interesting to note that children who sustain burns or scalds often appear to come from homes with several other young brothers and sisters, so that the mother is over-worked and unable to give much supervision. This also seems to be one of the reasons why many of these patients are still used to drinking from the bottle, well after the usual age. This possibility should always be kept in mind if there is difficulty in getting a young child to drink.

Children nursed by the exposure method often miss their usual coverings at first and if cold, can be covered by sterile towels and wear sterilized bootees and mittens. Little girls enjoy wearing pretty hair ribbons even if this is the only 'clothing' they are allowed. The young patients soon get used to their nakedness and although they may at first feel cold when transferred to the open ward they then often dislike being dressed.

Consideration for the mental welfare of the parents is as important as for the child. Parents often blame themselves in some way for the accident and some time may have to be spent with anxious parents outlining the treatment, the probable outcome of the illness and the degree of scarring and length of hospitalization to be expected. Parents of newly admitted children should be encouraged to speak to those of convalescent patients as they may be able to give them comfort from their own experiences.

Further reading

BLACK, J. A. (1979) *Paediatric Emergencies*. London: Butterworth.

JACKSON, R. H. (1977) *Children, the Environment and Accidents*. London: Pitman Medical.

MARKS, R. & SAMMAN, P. D. (1977) *Dermatology*. London: Heinemann Medical.

PEGUM, J. S. & BAKER, H. (1979) *Dermatology*, 3rd edn. London: Baillière Tindall.

VERBOV, J. (1979) *Modern Topics in Paediatric Dermatology*. London: Heinemann Medical.

14 Muscle, bones and joints

MUSCULAR DYSTROPHIES (MYOPATHIES)

A number of variants of the myopathies exist which all have the characteristics of progressive, degenerative changes in the muscle fibres, leading to wasting and weakness. The nerves are not affected in this group and there are neither sensory changes nor paralysis. The diseases are often hereditary and familial and usually lead to early death due to intercurrent infection such as pneumonia. A proportion of children with muscular dystrophy are mentally handicapped but the majority are of normal intelligence.

The various types of myopathies affect different muscle groups in particular, causing degenerative changes in the muscle fibres and their replacement by connective tissue and fat. Whole groups of muscles may thus be weakened and although the process may be a very slow one, it is always progressive and the patient eventually becomes completely incapacitated and crippled.

Diagnosis

Diagnosis is confirmed by electromyography, by which means the changes can be differentiated from those in other diseases of muscles. The destruction of muscle causes excretion of creatinine in the urine.

Pseudohypertrophic muscular dystrophy

The most common of the myopathies in childhood is

pseudohypertrophic muscular dystrophy so called because of the enlargement of certain muscles in this condition.

Signs and symptoms

The child may be normal up to school age but gradually it is noticed that he tires easily, that he prefers to sit about rather than play with other children, and finds it difficult to walk up stairs without the help of the banister. The gait becomes unstable and he is easily pushed over in play. The muscles of the shoulder girdle may become so weak that the child cannot raise his arms above his head and when the doctor places his hands underneath the arms to lift the patient, the child literally slips through his hands.

Weakness of the muscles of the pelvic girdle and the spine lead to kyphosis and lordosis. The gait is waddling at first and later becomes impossible. When the child tries to raise himself from the lying position, he first has to roll on to his front and then raise himself onto his hands and knees; by gradually moving one hand after the other up his legs and above his knees he eventually succeeds in raising himself to the upright position. This manoeuvre is very characteristic of the disease.

As the muscular weakness progresses the child becomes bedridden and deformities through contractions develop.

Treatment

Treatment aims at preventing crippling and wasting by massage and exercises. Movement should be encouraged as disuse leads to more rapid wasting. Pneumonia usually causes death after a few years.

Other types of the myopathies

These affect specific muscle groups in particular. The rate of progress may vary greatly and in spite of crippling the patient may survive into middle age. The more common varieties are the facioscapulohumeral type and myotonia congenita. As the name implies, the muscles affected in the facioscapulohumeral type, are those of the face, arms and shoulder girdle. The first signs may be difficulty in sucking and in closing the eyes completely. The handicap is, as a rule, slight and a fairly normal existence is possible. Myotonia congenita causes voluntary muscles to go into protracted contractions followed by slow relaxation. Muscle biopsy shows enlargement and thickening of muscle fibres. Muscle biopsy and electromyography are usually carried out to confirm diagnosis as the changes in the electrical activity in the muscle and those in the structure of the muscle are characteristic of the various types of the disease.

Genetic counselling should be offered to all parents considering enlarging their family.

TORTICOLLIS (WRY NECK)

Torticollis may be present from birth or arise later in life caused by diseases such as inflamed glands in the neck, tuberculosis of the cervical spine and paralysis. Occasionally the cause is psychological.

The postural changes are characteristic and include rotation of the head to one side with head flexion and a raising of the shoulder on the other. If allowed to persist, the angle at which the head is constantly held causes visual disturbances.

Treatment

This depends on the child's age and on the underlying cause. In infants, stretching and passive exercises should be carried out several times daily and correct posture maintained by means of sandbags and possibly a cap and light harness made of 12-mm webbing. Collars made of corrugated paper covered with a piece of soft material, Perspex splints, and supports and collars made from polystyrene are used to keep the head in an over-corrected position. In resistant cases, subcutaneous or open tenotomy may have to be carried out to lengthen the sternomastoid muscle. Post-operative over-correction is maintained for some time by one of the methods given above.

PERTHES' DISEASE

Osteochondritis is a fairly common abnormality of growth and development of the epiphyses in children. The most common of the diseases in this group is Perthes' disease. This disease affects boys more frequently than girls and develops between the ages of 5–10 years. It is usually unilateral.

The cause is a disturbance in the blood supply to the epiphysis, which leads to deformity of the epiphysial plate and in the later stages, if untreated, to collapse of the head of the femur and arrest of the development of the epiphysis.

Examination reveals that the range of movement is limited in all directions. Changes may not show up on radiographs for some time; after a while there may be wasting of the leg and in some cases shortening. The latter is due to collapse of the head and later premature epiphysial arrest. The disease takes a long course, the average time from onset to final healing is 4 years.

Treatment

There are two distinct approaches to the treatment of Perthes' disease. Some surgeons consider that prolonged immobilization with traction is required to prevent osteo-arthritis in later life. Others believe that once the early stage of muscle spasm is passed, ambulation with the aid of crutches is all that is required. If the disease process affects the entire femoral head osteotomy may be necessary. To avoid the effects of prolonged hospitalization these children, where possible, should be cared for at home with the support of the community nursing services.

Nursing management

Those children who are treated by bed-rest combined with traction and splinting, and those with calipers, have to be given special care of skin and pressure areas to prevent soreness. With the surgeon's permission groin and any other straps should be released twice daily and the skin washed, carefully dried and kept healthy by applying powder and zinc and castor oil cream (with or without the addition of compound of tincture of benzoin, sufficient to colour the cream light brown) and padding with a layer of lint or polyurethane.

General muscle tone should be maintained by giving daily massage and exercises. As the stay in hospital may extend over several weeks, schooling and play activities should be made available and whenever possible outings or a week-end visit home should be arranged.

Prognosis

The prognosis is excellent provided adequate early treatment is given but late cases may develop severe arthritis when they grow older.

CONGENITAL DISLOCATION OF THE HIP JOINT

Children with congenital dislocation of the hip joint have an abnormally shallow acetabulum which causes the femoral head to be displaced upwards and backwards when the child begins to put weight upon the limb. The neck of the femur may be shortened and the capsule becomes stretched. Sometimes the femoral head lies outside the acetabulum at the time of birth. As the child walks she dips on the affected side or has a waddling gait if the dislocation is a bilateral one. Because the pelvis is tipped forward, lordosis develops.

Congenital dislocation of the hip joint is a fairly common condition. Successful treatment depends on an early assessment and this should not be delayed beyond the first week of life.

The abnormality occurs most in girls; the condition runs in families and although usually present at birth it is often not noticed until the child begins to walk. The dislocation may be unilateral or bilateral and it may be partial or complete.

Signs and symptoms

The observant nurse may notice that one leg is shorter than the other and that the perineum is wider than usual. A telescoping movement of the leg may be possible. When the baby lies prone, the gluteal crease on the affected side is higher than that on the good side and the buttocks may be flattened.

When the baby is being medically examined she is placed on her back with the legs towards the examining doctor with hips and knees flexed at right angles. The middle finger of each hand is placed over the great trochanter while the flexed leg is contained in the palm of the hand and the thumb on the inner side of the thigh opposite the lesser trochanter. Keeping the legs flexed at 45° abduction the middle finger of each hand is pressed on the great trochanter to test whether or not the femoral head can be lifted into the acetabulum. If the test is positive, a click will be heard. This is known as the Ortolani sign.

Not in all cases in which the test is positive will treatment be necessary. An experienced orthopaedic surgeon must however be asked to see the baby without delay.

Treatment

Treatment should be started as soon as the condition has been recognized, as its duration and success depend on the age of the child. In very young babies a double nappy may give sufficient abduction to provide effective treatment. In more severe cases a harness splint may be used to maintain continuously the abducted position of the hips.

Older children may be placed on a special abduction frame and skin traction is applied to bring the head of the femur into position opposite the acetabulum. The legs are gradually abducted at intervals of 2 or 3 days to allow for gradual stretching of the muscles. When both legs have been abducted to right angles to the trunk (Fig. 47), the child is taken to the theatre.

Tenotomies may be necessary to obtain a fully abducted position of the hip joints in children over 18 months of age.

Two different methods of treatment are commonly used, depending on the age of the child, radiograph appearance and the surgeon's wishes:

1. The dislocation is reduced and the legs rotated to bring the femoral head into the acetabulum. The legs are fixed externally rotated and in full abduction with the knees flexed at right angles to the femora. A so-called '*frog plaster*' is applied, which reaches from the nipple line to the ankles.

2. The dislocation is reduced, the femora internally rotated and the legs fully abducted from the knees downward. A plaster, reaching from the groins to the ankles enable the child to move freely in the hip joint while maintaining flexion and extension. A wooden cross-bar is incorporated into the plaster from one knee across to the other: this is called a *Batchelor plaster*. After a time the child learns to move about and even to 'walk' on her knees.

In either case treatment has to be continued for a year to 18 months and during that time the child may be discharged home and brought back for changes of plaster at intervals of

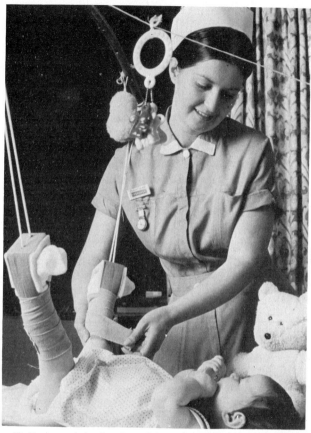

Fig. 47. Nurse renewing bandages following daily inspection of skin for child on hoop traction.

approximately 3 months. Occasionally neither of these methods is successful and open reduction and rotation osteotomy to correct the angle of the femur on the hip may be necessary. This would not be done until the baby is at least 1 year old. In very persistent cases shelf operation, acetabuloplasty, is performed to deepen the acetabulum, and a hip spica applied.

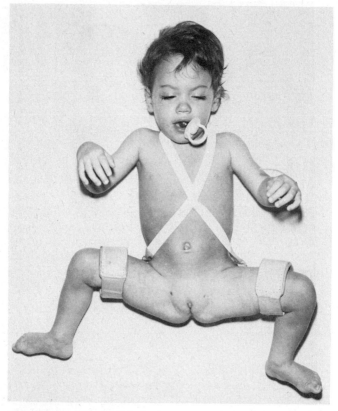

Fig. 48. Child with a congenitally dislocated hip with hip joints abducted in a Denis Browne harness.

During the stage of abduction the child suffers consider-ble discomfort and frustration due to the immobility and her position on the frame. A great deal of individual attention, occupation and visiting all help to comfort the child. In the initial stages sedatives should be given gener-ously. The nurse will have to use much patience and imagination to get the child to take fluids and food in this position and to teach her to pass urine and faeces without unduly soiling the padding of the frame. The bandages are taken off the legs daily and the skin inspected for reactions to strapping. They are washed and powdered before reapplying the bandages. The frame padding or plaster can be protected by thin plastic sheeting or waterproof adhesive tape.

Nursing management following manipulation and application of plaster

Nursing action

Plaster is exposed to allow for drying naturally. Patient turned 2–4-hourly.

Turn, using palms of hands only whilst plaster is still damp.

Observe toes for signs of plaster being too tight.

Apply bootees and mittens.

Support arms and feet with pillows.

Observe for pressure sores where child uses joints to move himself.

Adjust child's position to allow participation with surroundings. When plaster is dry the child can be taken for walks in a twin pushchair.

Provide suitable play activities.

Observe for the indications of plaster sores (restlessness, itching, fretfulness and slight rise in temperature).

Explanation

Drying plaster quickly causes cracking. Allow for drying of plaster back and front.

Avoids indentation of plaster which weakens it.

Tight plaster will obstruct blood supply (on digital pressure skin should flush quickly.

Extremities become cold quickly.

Can cause discomfort.

Elbows and heels become red and sore.

Child will become frustrated and irritable if isolated by position.

To encourage normal development and allay boredom.

The signs appear as the sore develops. Once the sores are established pain disappears. There may then be staining of the plaster.

The child is usually sent home and only readmitted for change of plaster and reassessment at intervals of 2–3 months. The mother is taught how to keep the plaster clean and to provide all care for her child. Before discharge home the family health visitor should be informed in order to provide on-going support and counselling to the mother and the family.

Treatment to continue over a period of 1–2 years depending in part on the age of the child, as the longer the condition has been left untreated the more difficult is successful treatment. When the plaster is eventually omitted, the child is at first allowed the freedom of the bed. Daily physiotherapy is given and after about 3 weeks, if X-ray appearance is satisfactory, the child is allowed to start weight-bearing. In early, successful cases walking should be normal and a complete, permanent cure can be expected.

TALIPES

Talipes (Fig. 49) may occur on one or both sides and is often associated with other congenital abnormalities such as spina bifida. There are variants in severity and in the type of deformity. Usually several joints of the foot are involved, often causing inversion of the forefoot, internal rotation of the tibia and plantar flexion of the ankle joint. There are four types, and any may be seen in varying degrees of severity.

1. *Talipes equinovarus* (*clubfoot*). The deformity consists of inversion (turning in) of the forefoot, internal rotation of the tibia and plantar flexion of the ankle joint.

2. *Congenital talipes calcaneovalgus*. The deformity consists of eversion (turning out) of the foot and dorsiflexion at the ankle joint. The tendon Achillis is lengthened. This deformity is less severe and yields more easily to treatment

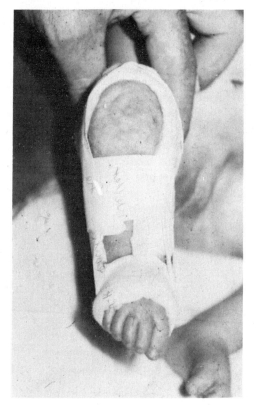

Fig. 49. Talipes equinovarus foot strapped in the correct position.

than the equinovarus deformity. In mild cases it may be sufficient for the mother to stretch the foot into equinus and varus position several times before each feed. She will also have to do this in cases which require surgery.

3. *Talipes equinovalgus.* In this deformity there is eversion and plantar flexion.

4. *Taliper calcaneovarus.* In this deformity there is inversion and dorsiflexion.

The two last-mentioned deformities are usually seen in children with paralysis and/or cerebral palsy.

Treatment of talipes equinovarus

This should be commenced within 36 hours of birth and its success depends greatly on the promptness with which it is started. The foot is manipulated manually until the little toe touches the peroneal surface of the leg. The over-corrected position is maintained by adhesive strapping, splints, Plaster of Paris or special Denis Browne boots. Manipulation is repeated weekly at first. Kicking and standing on the splints when the child is old enough are encouraged as this helps to develop the leg muscles.

Manipulation often causes reactionary swelling and as treatment is often given in the out-patient department full instructions to bring her baby back if there is reason for concern, should be given to the mother, in the same way as would be done in cases of fractures treated by Plaster of Paris.

If treated from birth, correction may be complete by the age of 6 months or a year but a special night boot is usually worn for another year or two. Occasionally the outside of the shoe heel is raised or an inside iron with a 'T' strap fixed to the shoes when the baby starts to walk.

Long-term care

Cases treated less promptly may need many years of treatment, and cure may not be permanent. Parents are usually very pleased with the initial improvement and it may be difficult to impress on them the importance of continuing treatment for a number of years. Sometimes manipulation, stretching and splinting fail and operation becomes necessary. This may be either open or closed tenotomy, or, as a last resort, Steindler's operation or triple arthrodesis.

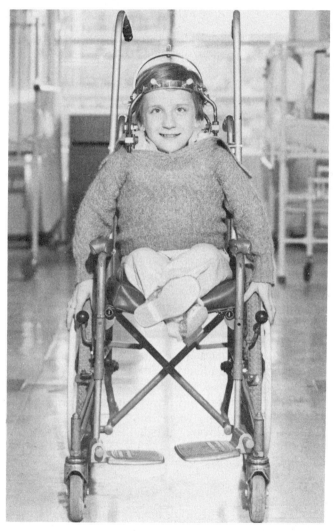

Fig. 50. Mobile with the aid of a wheelchair.

OSTEOMYELITIS

Osteomyelitis is an infection causing acute inflammation beneath the periosteum, resulting in an abscess and sequestrum formation (death of the bone).

The disease attacks children between the ages of 2 and 12 years, although babies in the neonatal period may be affected. The femur, humerus, clavicle and maxilla are common sites of infection and there may be evidence of a recent knock or injury. There is frequently a history of infected tonsils, boils or septic spots and the causative organism is often the staphylococcus.

Signs and symptoms

The onset may be acute with hyperpyrexia, tachycardia, headaches, rigor, toxaemia or septicaemia, but at times it can be quite insidious. Infants appear to have little pain, but the general disturbances include vomiting and diarrhoea, causing dehydration, In older children pain can be very severe until tension subsides following treatment with antibiotics which reduce the infection.

The limb is held immobilized in a relaxed position and occasionally the condition may be mistaken for some form of paralysis. Any handling is deeply resented. The skin over the affected area may be found to be red, shiny and hot, although it may take a day or two for the inflammation to become obvious. The white cell count is high (mainly polymorphonuclear cells) and blood culture is sometimes positive. X-ray appearance is rarely abnormal before the second or third week.

Treatment

Large doses of antibiotics together with immobilization, may bring about a cure, but sometimes the child does not respond well. Analgesia should be given whenever needed.

The usual antibiotics in this case are penicillin, kanamycin and cloxacillin, given by injection. Surgery may become necessary to either drain an abscess that has formed, or to remove damaged bone.

Nursing management

As there may be exquisite pain, jarring of the bed must be avoided and for that reason the bed should be situated in a corner of the ward in the acute stage. Temperature, pulse and respirations are taken every 4 hours and fluid intake and output charts kept up to date. Abundant fluids are given and as the child is often negative and reluctant to drink, it is important to vary the drinks by using different flavours and by alternating hot and cold drinks.

Once the fever has subsided, a nourishing, high protein diet is given to build up the child's general health. Small pillows, sand-bags and air rings should be used to ensure a comfortable position and rest for the affected part.

Every effort should be made to maintain as many of the child's normal activities as possible, e.g. schooling and play activities.

N.B. In the presence of any draining wound the child should be isolated and nursed with full barrier precautions.

SYNDACTYLY

Syndactyly or webbing of the digits of the hands and feet may be partial or complete. The underlying bones and joints may be normal, or sections may be missing or fused. The plastic surgeon may be able to separate the digits and to give the hand an aesthetically good appearance, without much difficulty. Or it may be necessary to utilize one of the fingers as a thumb by transplanting muscles in such a way as to bring one digit into apposition to the others to make gripping possible. Occasionally skin grafting is undertaken to supply skin for the surfaces between the divided digits.

In looking after these patients post-operatively it is important to watch for signs of impaired circulation, sometimes a difficult task as the entire hand or foot may be covered in a tight crêpe bandage.

OSTEOGENESIS IMPERFECTA
(FRAGILITAS OSSIUM)

As the name suggests, the bones in fragilitas ossium are fragile and fractures occur on the least provocation. There are two main types of the disease. In the antenatal variety most of the bones of the fetal skull and skeleton have sustained fractures before birth. Callus formation causes the bones to be thickened and deformed. Babies with this complaint have markedly blue sclerotics. The condition is familial and severe cases become seriously handicapped, while others die at birth due to fractures occurring during labour.

In the second variety the fractures occur mostly after the first year of life. The bones are porous and the teeth translucent. Although the fractures heal rapidly, deformities inevitably result and these children lead sheltered lives with schooling frequently interrupted by treatment or admissions to hospital. Occasionally the condition improves at puberty. Neither the cause nor any effective treatment are known.

CORRECTION OF DEFORMITIES CAUSED
BY PARALYSIS

The abnormal and imbalanced pulls of certain muscle groups against others weakened by paralysis can cause severe and progressive deformities in the growing child. Surgical treatment is often necessary to prevent deformity and to stabilize joints and so to improve function. The results of infantile paralysis, congenital abnormalities of the spine (e.g. myelomeningocele) and cerebral palsy are examples.

Corrective operations include transplantation of tendons in the leg or foot. This transplantation aims at counteracting an abnormal pull from a group of healthy muscles which would lead to deformity. Transplantation of the tendons of the hamstring muscles, for instance to the back of the femur, may enable a child with spastic paralysis to straighten his knees and to walk almost normally.

Tenotomy may be performed to lengthen certain tendons, e.g. a contracted Achilles tendon in the child with cerebral palsy in order to promote mobility.

Further reading

BRUNNER, L. S. & SUDDARTH, D. S. (1981) *The Lippincott Manual of Paediatric Nursing*. London: Harper & Row.

LLOYD-ROBERTS, G. C. & RATLIFF, A. H. C. (1978) *Hip Disorders in Children*. London: Butterworth.

POWELL, M. (1982) *Orthopaedic Nursing & Rehabilitation*, 8th edn. London: Churchill Livingstone.

ROAF, R. & HODKINSON, L. J. (1980) *Textbook of Orthopaedic Nursing*, 3rd edn. Oxford: Blackwell Scientific.

15 Disorders involving the genitourinary system

The kidney excretes waste products of metabolism, and acts as a filter and reabsorbs certain substances necessary to the body. A nurse who understands the importance of any abnormalities in the urine and who uses her powers of observation to the full should not find the toilet round a boring routine but will appreciate her responsibility in this respect. Her careful reporting may help the physician who relies on the accuracy of her reports and tests.

Observations should be recorded clearly and accurately on the patient's chart and abbreviations should be avoided as they may easily lead to misinterpretations or misunderstandings.

Methods of collecting clean and ordinary specimens of urine
Even newborn babies may show signs of renal damage due to abnormalities present in utero, e.g. back pressure caused by inadequate relaxation of the bladder neck or sphincter or inadequate muscle action in the bladder wall or ureters. Such damage is usually irreversible.

Infection in infancy, caused by ascending bacterial invasion or by deformities such as double ureters, neurogenic bladder, horseshoe kidney, etc., may lead to permanent renal damage in later life unless treated at the earliest possible moment. Careful collection of urine for examination is therefore of very great importance.

Accurate measurement of the urinary output and drainage is of paramount importance as it may be an aid to

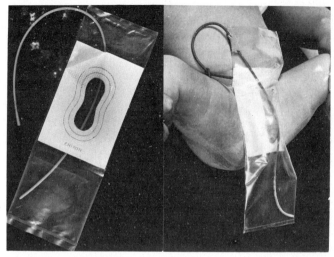

Fig. 51. Urine collecting bag (*left*), in position (*right*). The bag may be used for either boys or girls for obtaining single specimens, or for 24-hour collections.

diagnosis and lead to the prevention of serious complications. Where appropriate the nurse should state whether the urine came from a nephrostomy, perineal or suprapubic or urethral catheter or if it was passed normally per urethram.

It may be difficult to collect urine from babies and toddlers. The container should be of appropriate size for the amount of urine collected (e.g. 10-ml bottles are quite adequate for babies). Special plastic urine collecting bags may be used both for boys and girls (Fig. 51). Where these are not available the following techniques can be used:

Baby boys. Urine may be collected by strapping a test tube or Paul's tubing to the penis. If the specimen is for bacteriological investigation, an aseptic technique should be used. A tray with receivers and sterile cotton wool swabs, saline or a mild antiseptic solution, such as 1% cetrimide, a sterile test tube or Paul's tubing, and four lengths of 6 mm (¼ in.) strapping is required. The penis is well cleaned, where possible the foreskin retracted and the glans gently swabbed before fixing the tube in position. Paul's tubing, previously sterilized, is easy to use and very effective.

Baby girls. Baby girls present a much more difficult problem. It may be advisable to wash and swab the buttocks and genitalia carefully before commencing a feed and then to sit the baby on a sterile receiver while she is feeding. Babies often pass urine during a feed.

Alternatively, a sterile receiver may be placed inside a well fitting air-ring and the baby nursed sitting upright over the opening.

Catheterization

Catheterization in young children should be avoided whenever possible. Sometimes catheterization may have to be carried out for diagnostic purposes, to relieve retention of urine, and in certain post-operative cases.

Basically the requirements are the same for children as for adults. It is, however, essential to have at least one assistant or whenever possible the mother present, to ensure that the child maintains the correct position without struggling and who can reassure and talk to the child.

Little girls should have their buttocks raised on a sand bag or rolled towel. When the buttocks are thus elevated the catheter should be directed downwards rather than at right angles to the perineum, as it would be with an adult. As the urethra is short urine should be obtained after passing only 2.5–5 cm (1–2 in.) of the catheter. It is important to wash the groins, thighs and genitalia with soap and water before starting the actual catheterization. When the procedure is completed the surrounding skin should be carefully dried. A pot or bedpan should be offered as catheterization leaves the patient with a feeling of irritation and an apparent desire to pass urine.

Suprapubic aspiration in order to obtain sterile urine specimens is often carried out instead of catheterization. This procedure is performed by a doctor with a fine needle and syringe. By this means the specimen obtained is not contaminated with other organisms, and there is less likelihood of introducing infection into the bladder.

Mid-stream specimens

With older children, capable of cooperation and control in passing urine, this method can replace catheterization in many cases. After cleaning the genital area in the method described above, the child is asked to pass some urine in order to flush the urethra. After approximately 30 g (1 oz) has been passed the stream is interrupted and the remaining urine collected in a sterile container with clear indication that the specimen was a mid-stream one.

Twenty-four-hour specimens. To estimate accurately the volume of urine passed in 24 hours, the following procedure is adopted.

The patient is asked to empty the bladder at 08.00 hours and this urine is discarded. All urine is passed in the following 24 hours is then collected. The patient is asked to pass urine at 07.55 hours the following day and this specimen is added to the total collected.

Retention of urine

This, irrespective of the cause, may produce restlessness in unconscious patients and may disturb sleep. Simple nursing measures may relieve retention. The nurse can partly fill the pot or bedpan with warm water, sit the patient in a warm bath, allow small boys to stand up while using a bottle, and run a nearby tap. Such nursing attention is infinitely worthwhile and may make painful, complicated measures such as catheterization unnecessary.

Investigations of the Urinary Tract

Intravenous pyelography

Intravenous pyelograms are done to outline the urinary tract and demonstrate the efficiency of renal function. Fluids are withheld for the 6 hours preceding the test but dry foods may be given.

A straight radiograph is taken first, in order to ascertain that no gases will obscure the picture. If this is satisfactory a radio-opaque dye is then injected into a vein. In most cases the median basilic vein is chosen for the injection but with babies it may be necessary to use another vein if possible, but occasionally it is necessary for the medium to be subcutaneously combined with hyaluronidase in order to speed up and facilitate absorption. The dye is rapidly excreted by the urinary tract.

N.B. *Iodine sensitivity*. A test dose of 1 ml is injected intravenously. If no reaction occurs in 1 minute the full dose of the opaque medium can be given. *Sensitivity reaction*: nausea, vomiting, urticaria, flushing and restlessness.

Immediately after the injection the child is given a 'fizzy drink' or an infant is given a feed. This allows for the demonstration of the left kidney on X-ray behind the gas bubble formed in the stomach.

Serial pictures are taken, usually at 3, 8, 15 and 30 minutes after the injection and the progress of the dye is watched. Any abnormalities in the filling of the renal tract or in excretion are demonstrated on the radiograph.

Micturating cystogram

Cooperation will be needed from the older child during

this procedure, so the nurse should carefully explain what is involved prior to catheterization. If the mother is accompanying the child, she too should clearly understand the procedure. A small child may have the examination carried out under a general anaesthetic. The child is usually catheterized in the ward, before transfer to the X-ray department. Following introduction of the contrast medium through the catheter, this is then removed and the child encouraged to pass urine. As the bladder contracts X-rays are taken. If the cystogram is being carried out under a general anaesthetic, suprapubic pressure is needed to empty the bladder.

Cystoscopy

Cystoscopy is exactly the same as with adults except that children are given a light anaesthetic. Cystoscopy is usually done to examine the bladder, urethra, and ureteric openings into the bladder for congenital abnormalities.

Retrograde pyelography

Retrograde pyelography is sometimes needed to ascertain further evidence, particularly if, due to poor renal function, the intravenous pyelogram has failed to yield adequate information.

For this procedure a lighter anaesthetic has to be given but otherwise preparation is the same as for intravenous pyelogram, and the procedure is similar to that used in adults.

Cystography

Cystography may be done in order to determine the capacity and outline of the bladder or to demonstrate the presence of urethral valves and vesico-ureteric reflux.

Renal biopsy

Renal biopsy is carried out under a general anaesthetic as

an aid to the assessment and progress of renal tissue, particularly for those children suffering from nephritis or nephrosis. It may also be performed following a kidney transplant.

Following return to the ward after the procedure, nursing care should monitor the following:

Nursing action	Explanation
Pulse and blood pressure.	Any increase may indicate haemorrhage into the renal tissue.
All urine passed is measured and examined for blood.	Some haematuria is usually present for 24 hours. If persistent or excessive, report to doctor.
Pain related to site of puncture, backache and dysuria.	Some discomfort expected initially, prescribed analgesia should be given. If persistent or excessive, report to doctor. May indicate renal damage.
Puncture site should be left exposed to observe for swelling, discolouration and haemorrhage.	Report any change. May indicate damage to other tissues or renal haemorrhage.

Renal function tests

Urea clearance test

A comparison is made between the amount of urea present in the circulation and urine respectively. The test demonstrates the extent of healthily functioning substance in the kidney, following disease.

Urea concentration test

This is a test of the kidneys' ability to excrete urea, one of the end products of protein metabolism. The child has nothing to eat or drink for 12 hours (usually overnight) before the test.

Urine is then collected, following which a dose of urea is given. A further 3 specimens of urine are collected at hourly intervals.

Ureatine clearance test

A 24-hour collection of urine is commenced. During this period a specimen of blood is obtained. The laboratory staff will need to know the child's age, sex, height and weight in order to assess glomerular function in the excretion of ureatine, a breakdown product of protein metabolism.

ACUTE PYELONEPHRITIS (PYELITIS)

This is essentially an infection of the renal parenchyma and the pelvis of the kidney. The disease is a very common one in childhood, affecting girls rather more often than boys and it occurs frequently in young infants.

Mode of infection

The infection may reach the kidneys via the blood stream, from the bowel via the lymphatic system or as an ascending infection from the bladder and urethra. In many cases the infection is caused by a malformation in the urinary tract, such as a kink in one of the ureters which causes the urine to be dammed back, to stagnate and to become infected.

In about 70% of cases the causative organism is the *Escherichia coli* (bacterium), but streptococcal and staphylococcal infections also occur.

Signs and symptoms

As a rule, the onset of the disease is a very sudden one. One of the earliest symptoms is vomiting, soon followed by a rise in temperature to between 39.4° and 40.6°C (103°–105°F); rigors and meningism are common. The child is pale and ashen in colour, with flushed cheeks and dark rings round the eyes. She is irritable and there are signs that she is suffering from spasmodic, colicky pain, which is a constant feature. With young babies diarrhoea occurs and this together with the vomiting soon causes dehydration. The urine is scanty, strongly acid and may have a curious fishy smell. The tongue is dry and thirst is marked. If old enough to do so the patient complains of dysuria.

Investigations

Examination of a clean specimen of fresh urine under the microscope will reveal the presence of pus cells, albumin and organisms. The prognosis is as a rule a good one, recovery taking place in 3 days to a week. Recurrent cases are often due to malformations in the urinary tract and therefore X-ray investigations are carried out. The prognosis depends on the underlying cause.

Nursing care

The nursing care in the case of an attack of pyelitis is mostly symptomatic. In order to reduce the temperature, the bedclothes are cradled and a fan may be used to cool and circulate the air. Tepid sponging is soothing but must not be done without medical permission. If the patient is incontinent the buttocks should be washed frequently as the acid urine is liable to excoriate the skin. Zinc and castor oil cream should be applied. The mouth easily gets dry and dirty, and careful mouth toilet is essential.

Temperature, pulse and respirations are taken and recorded 4-hourly and a strict intake and output record is important. If vomiting persists and dehydration becomes marked, fluids may have to be given intravenously.

Drugs

According to the sensitivity of the causative organism, various drugs such as sulphonamides and nitrofurantoin are administered.

Diet

In the majority of cases the patient should be given liberal amounts of fluids especially while on sulphonamide therapy. For babies, milk is withheld as long as vomiting persists. Once the acute stage of the illness is passed, children quickly regain their appetite and no special diets need be given.

NEPHRITIS

A variety of classifications of nephritis have been used in the past, but the term nephritis is now used for those conditions in which inflammatory changes predominate in the renal substance. Nephrosis or nephrotic syndrome is characterized by degenerative changes in the renal tubules. Sometimes it is difficult to draw a distinction between the two conditions and in the sub-acute phase the term 'nephrotic-nephritis' may be used.

Table 8. Comparison between nephritis and nephrotic syndrome

	Nephritis	Nephrotic syndrome
Onset	Very sudden	Insidious
Cause	Streptococcal infection 10–14 days previously in 75% of cases	Unknown in many cases, in others associated with renal disease
Age	Commonly 3–8 years, rarely in infancy	All ages
Haematuria	Present	Rarely present
Proteinuria	Moderate degree	Considerable
Urinary output	Diminished	Variable
Oedema	Of short duration if it occurs	Persistent
Blood pressure	Raised at onset	Usually normal
Diet	Restricted protein, low salt if oedema present	High protein, low salt

Nephritis

Acute post streptococcal glomerulonephritis; acute haemorrhagic nephritis.

Definition

A disease of sudden onset, usually following a streptococcal infection (most commonly tonsillitis) 10–14 days prior to onset of haematuria, hypertension and acute renal inflammation.

Pathology

Both kidneys are affected, but are of normal size. Microscopical appearance shows minute haemorrhages blocking the glomeruli which means that the filtering capacity of the kidneys is interfered with; small areas of necrosis may also be seen.

Age

Affects most commonly the age group 3–8 years; rarely in infancy.

Clinical presentation

Haematuria is often the presenting symptom, it may be very obvious or only minimal giving a 'smoky' appearance to the urine. This may last for a few days or for many weeks. Urinary output at onset of the disease is usually diminished. The child appears 'off colour', disinterested in his normal play activities and very lethargic. Headache and vomiting frequently occur at onset of the disease. Oedema is common, and is especially noted in the eyelids and the pendant parts, but is of short duration. It is associated with an increase in weight. In cases of streptococcal infection the antistreptolysin titre is raised. The temperature is elevated and the blood pressure may remain normal but more commonly it will also be raised.

Investigations

These will include daily ward tests of urine, quantitative daily albumin estimations may also be recorded. Laboratory examinations of the urine to detect the presence of cells and casts will be required at frequent intervals, but less often once the haematuria has disappeared. As the kidney cannot clear the waste products in the normal way, the blood urea level may rise about 7.47 mmol/litre (45 mg/100 ml) or more, and creatinine and phosphorus levels are also higher than usual. Culture of throat swabs and a full blood count will also be made. X-ray of the sinuses and examination of the tonsils and teeth are carried out in order to discover any foci of infection.

Treatment

Diet, rest and nursing care are the main forms of treatment. Penicillin may be prescribed for any latent streptococcal infection. Anaemia is treated with iron therapy. Sulphonamides may be ordered.

Nursing care

Children suffering from nephritis are kept on bed rest, until urinary output and blood pressure are normal, and the haematuria has subsided. The child should be kept warm, and nursed in a semi-recumbent position so that he is comfortable, resting, and yet able to watch the life of the ward around him. A daily blanket bath is given and the pressure areas treated 4-hourly. Mouth care is particularly important, and is carried out frequently. If constipation is troublesome a mild aperient may be given.

The nurse should make time to play and read with her patient in order to relieve the monotony of bed rest. Parental visiting should be enouraged to enable the child to maintain his family contacts, and to adjust to hospitalization. Later, the child will be able to take part in the activities of the hospital school.

Obervations

1. Temperature, pulse and respiration are recorded 4-hourly initially as any change may be the first indication of complications developing, e.g. further infection.

2. Fluid intake and output should be recorded with accuracy.

3. Frequent recordings of the child's weight are made; it is most useful to chart this as a graph to show progress, as it is a good guide to the amount of oedema present.

4. Blood pressure readings are taken twice daily initially, then less frequently if good progress is made. Any rise in the blood pressure readings must be reported immediately.

5. The appearance of an early morning specimen of urine should be noted daily.

6. Note of the child's general appearance must also be made, e.g. how he looks and if he appears to be more, or less, interested in his surroundings. Any observation of twitching of the limbs should be reported immediately as this may be an indication that hypertensive encephalopathy, a serious complication, is developing.

Diet

In order to rest the kidneys the fluid intake is usually restricted during the initial phase; the amount allowed varies according to the child's weight.

Examples of the amount of fluid allowed in 24 hours

5 years	18 kg (40 lb)	Basic allowance	360 ml (12 oz)
10 years	30 kg (66 lb)	Basic allowance	480 ml (16 oz)

Added to the basic allowance would be an amount equal to the volume of urine passed during the previous 24 hours.

For the first 3 or 4 days the child's diet consists of fresh fruit drinks with added glucose. Orange juice should be avoided in view of its relatively high potassium content.

The nurse should remember that the child will enjoy variety, and hot drinks as well as cold should be offered to relieve the monotony of the fluid diet. When diuresis occurs a light diet is gradually introduced, the protein of which is restricted until the urine tests show an improvement in the cell count. While any oedema is present, salt intake too will be restricted.

Prognosis
1. The majority of cases are uncomplicated and usually resolve in about 6 weeks.
2. Rarely, hypertension may lead to cardiac failure and encephalopathy. A few patients progress into the nephrotic syndrome. If anuria develops the outlook is grave.

NEPHROSIS, NEPHROTIC SYNDROME (LIPOID NEPHROSIS, SUBACUTE NEPHRITIS)

Definition
This condition is manifested clinically by insidious onset of gross generalized oedema, and by proteinuria, associated with low plasma proteins.

Pathology
Both kidneys are affected and appear very pale and swollen.

Age
Pure nephrosis or lipoid nephrosis, starts in children below the age of 5 years. Nephrotic syndrome, associated with a variety of other kidney conditions is seen in older children.

Clinical presentation
The child appears irritable, listless and pale with no interest in food. Oedema affects the face, legs and abdomen

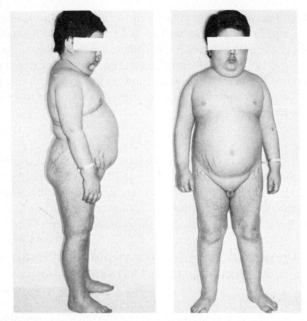

Fig. 52. A child with nephrotic syndrome who is also Cushingoid from the effect of over-treatment with steroids.

leading to weight gain. Urine output is reduced and proteinurea is present. Haematuria may occur and usually indicates a poor prognosis. Blood pressure initially is normal.

Investigations

Daily ward testing of urine and estimation of the amount of protein lost in the urine. Frequent laboratory examination of the urine for cells and casts, also culture for evidence of infection in the urine is required. Blood investigations needed will include a total blood picture, urea levels which are normal until the terminal stages, total plasma proteins which are low, serum cholesterol which is usually raised, and the ESR which may be elevated. Serum electrolytes should be estimated frequently. Renal biopsy may be performed to confirm the diagnosis if there is any doubt about this.

Drugs

Steroid therapy in the form of prednisone or prednisolone is of great value to the child with nephrosis; initially doses are high, the amount given being reduced after 10 days until a maintenance dose is reached to prevent the return of proteinuria. This maintenance dose may need to continue for as long as 6 months, but unfortunately relapses are common so that a return to higher dosages may be necessary. The long-term effect of steroids is to produce dwarfism, obesity and adrenal failure. The child receiving long-term steroids may need to receive antibiotics as a prophylactic measure as these children are especially prone to infection.

In steroid resistant cases, the diuretic chlorothiazide may be combined with spironolactone (Aldactone A) in a dosage of 25 mg four times daily. Potassium chloride should be given during therapy with chlorothiazide to prevent a potassium deficiency occurring. Cyclophosphamide (3 mg/kg) is sometimes combined with steroids for those children liable to relapse. The child and the parents should be warned that this drug may produce baldness, but that the hair will quickly grow again once the course of treatment has been completed. Meanwhile a wig can be worn if necessary.

A blood transfusion is given occasionally to correct anaemia and to improve the child's general condition.

Nursing care

The basic nursing care is the same as that for the child with nephritis, but as the oedema may be causing respiratory embarrassment the nurse will have to use her skills in making the patient comfortable with extra pillows. Support for the scrotum may be necessary if the patient is a boy. As the child with gross oedema will be unable to move much, conscientious care of the skin and pressure areas is important. Small pillows and bed cradles should be used to prevent foot drop and to take the weight of the bed clothes off the patient's limbs. An air ring may be valuable as an aid to comfort and to prevent pressure sores. The peripheral circulation is often poor and oedematous limbs may be cold and discoloured; warm blankets and woollen socks may help to keep the feet warm. Care must be taken to use hot-water bottles as the oedematous limbs are relatively insensitive, and burns could occur easily.

Because of the loss of gamma globulin together with oedema, there is a great tendency to infection and evidence of sepsis such as septic spots on the skin should be reported immediately.

Observations

Observations are the same as for the child with nephritis except that it is not usually necessary to record the blood pressure as frequently unless it is found to be raised.

Diet

As a great deal of protein is lost in the urine, a high protein diet is given as soon as the child is well enough to eat it. Estimations of the blood urea will act as a guide to tolerance of this regime; if the blood urea rises excessively it may be necessary to restrict protein intake. Restriction of salt to less than 2 g daily is also necessary while there is evidence of oedema. Paediatricians vary as to the need to restrict fluids, some allow 600 ml a day, others relate the fluid intake to the urinary output, while others do not restrict fluids at all.

Anorexia is frequently a problem, and the nurse needs to use skill and ingenuity to tempt the child's appetite by serving meals as attractively as possible. When a precise amount of protein is sent up from the diet kitchen the amount of food rejected should be recorded after every meal, so that the amount of protein refused can be accurately measured.

Prognosis

The long-term outlook is not good despite the use of steroids. Approximately 30% of patients die from complications, e.g. intercurrent infections or peritonitis. Some children after a variable period become symptom free, in others the oedema persists.

RENAL FAILURE

Renal failure occurs when the kidneys are unable to maintain regulation of the composition or the volume of the body fluids. With acute renal failure the child's condition deteriorates rapidly in a few days. The chronic form of renal failure may take several months. The main causes of renal failure are:

1. Shock associated with major injury or haemorrhage.
2. Burns involving more than 15% of the body surface.
3. Gastroenteritis resulting in severe dehydration.
4. Septicaemia.
5. Renal disease.
6. Obstructed urinary flow.
7. Mismatched transfusion, ingested poisons, anaphylactic shock.
8. Hypoxia in the neonatal period.

Signs and symptoms

The usual presenting symptom in acute renal failure is

oliguria, but occasionally the child will be observed to pass dilute urine in large quantities. Drowsiness, headache, loss of appetite, pallor, vomiting, sore dry mouth, pyrexia, diarrhoea and convulsions are all common and may occur simultaneously or at different times. Blood pressure and intracranial pressure are high and there may be visual disturbances and retinal haemorrhages. The pulse rate is rapid and the volume poor.

Treatment

Uraemic children are particularly prone to infection, and the appropriate antibiotics will be ordered. These may need to be given in reduced dosage, as some reach dangerous blood level concentrations if given in the normal amounts when the kidneys are not properly functioning, e.g. gentamycin, streptomycin, kanamycin and the sulphonamides. Intravenous fluids will be required for some children depending on the primary cause of the renal failure. For the severely anaemic child blood will be required and will usually be given as packed cells in order to avoid overloading the circulation. Peritoneal dialysis or haemodialysis is sometimes indicated if the child's condition continues to deteriorate and the blood urea level rises above 65 mmol/litre (400 mg/100 ml). Haemodialysis is the most effective method but requires special facilities that are not available in all units. For most children peritoneal dialysis is effective and can be used even in young children. Kidney transplant operations in children have now been carried out most successfully in a few specialized units. This offers a new life to these children but unfortunately there are not yet enough suitable donors and there are still many technical problems to overcome.

Nursing care

The aim of nursing care throughout this illness is to make

the child comfortable by anticipating needs, alleviating symptoms and providing the nurse's prescription of t.l.c. (Tender Loving Care).

Accurate records of the intake and output must be carefully maintained. The basic fluid intake should be totalled together with the output of the previous 24 hours and calculated to allow for insensible loss through the skin and lungs which the nurse should remember will be greater during a heatwave or if the child is pyrexial. Because of the poor kidney function only small amounts are allowed. An average daily fluid intake allowance would be:

Infants	12–15 ml/kg/24 hours.
Older children	10 ml/kg/24 hours.

The mouth will be dry and careful mouth toilet is essential. For the older child frequent mouth washes can be given providing he knows not to swallow any of the glycothymoline or whatever fluid is being used. Sucking fruit pastilles slowly, will also help to keep the mouth moist as well as providing extra calories. Adequate calories must be given in the diet to minimize further protein breakdown. A pleasantly flavoured glucose concentrate such as 'Hycal' (25 ml = 60 calories approx.) can be given. Some first-class protein will also need to be provided in the diet to prevent further breakdown of body protein and so increase the blood urea. Occasionally if the child is comatosed 'Aminosol' or 'Intralipid' will be given intravenously to meet essential nutrition requirements. Daily weight should be recorded ideally using a weighing bed, taking care that the bedclothes remain the same weight. Temperature, pulse and blood pressure readings should be recorded frequently and any changes reported.

Peritoneal dialysis

The procedure should be carefully explained to the child

before the treatment commences. The child should also empty his bladder and be weighed. A sedative may be required. Strict asepsis is observed throughout the procedure. The abdominal skin is cleaned and the doctor will infiltrate a local anaesthetic of 1% lignocaine into the skin midway between the umbilicus and symphysis pubis. A stab incision is made through which a 'Trocath' is introduced and a catheter is pushed gently into the pelvis and connected to the previously prepared dialysing set. The amount of dialysing fluid run in depends on the age and weight of each child. Small infants will accommodate 150–200 ml each run, but a child of 12 years may take as much as a litre. The first run is drained immediately but in subsequent cycles the fluid is allowed to remain in the peritoneal cavity for 30 minutes. Dialysis is used continuously until the plasma electrolytes are more or less normal. Throughout this procedure the nurse must observe the child most carefully, noting any difficulty in respiration, nausea or vomiting. Care should be taken to prevent kinking of the tubing. If the flow diminishes it can often be rectified by changing the child's position or repositioning the catheter. If the catheter becomes blocked, the doctor will need to syringe it through with heparinized saline, or replace it with a new one.

SURGICAL CONDITIONS OF THE
GENITO-URINARY TRACT

In childhood the majority of operations performed on the genito-urinary system are to correct congenital abnormalities. These are often the cause of recurrent urinary tract infections, colicky pain, and failure to thrive. In extreme, untreated cases, uraemia and death may result.

In investigations and treatments of the urinary tract the danger of ascending infection must constantly be borne in mind. Catheterization, the use of in-dwelling catheters, is only ordered if there is no other alternative. When drainage tubes are in use it is the task of the nurse to watch the tube carefully. Kinking or compression of the tube may lead to damming-back of urine and as a child is unlikely to voice his complaint it is the nurse's responsibility to appreciate that there is something wrong by noticing the patient's restlessness or by noticing an abnormal output of urine. Accurate measurement of the urinary drainage and output is more important if serious complications are to be prevented. Operations on bladder or kidney may result in bleeding and clot formation. Morphine may be given to lower blood pressure and relieve pain, and lavage may have to be employed to dissolve clots and prevent the child from straining in an attempt to pass the clot per urethram. At operations which may be expected to cause post-operative bleeding, the surgeon usually stitches a drainage tube into the wound, the substance of the kidney or the bladder to allow blood to escape. These tubes or drains call for careful nursing attention and vigilance.

Movement of the patient need not be restricted and change of position from side to side is helpful in promoting drainage and preventing chest complications.

Congenital abnormalities and their treatment

Agenesis of the kidney

Failure of development of the kidney is as a rule unilateral. In that case the other kidney may hypertrophy and take over the total renal function and no treatment is necessary. Bilateral agenesis is incompatible with survival beyond the neonatal period.

Horseshoe and double kidney

A horseshoe kidney is formed by the union of the lower

poles of the two kidneys, and may remain symptomless. The abnormality may be found accidentally in the course of a routine abdominal X-ray examination, or in other instances the child has recurrent urinary tract infections or attacks of pain and vomiting. A double kidney shows up plainly when pyelography is performed and it is often associated with double ureters. In long-standing cases hydronephrosis may develop. One of the ureters may have a kink or stenosis and if this is the cause of the recurrent infection or pain, it is removed.

Hydronephrosis and megaureter or hydroureter

Recurrent infections, obstructions and congenital abnormalities of urethra, ureters or renal pelvis may cause dilatation of one or both ureters or renal pelves. The patient suffers severe, recurrent pain and vomiting. The obstruction may be due to abnormally situated blood vessels which press on the ureters, stenosis of the ureter, ureteric or urethral valves, obstruction in the bladder neck and neurological causes. The obstruction may be unilateral or bilateral. If the cause of the obstruction can be removed, the ureters may regain their tone and return to a normal size. Nephrostomy and pyeloplasty are performed to relieve the condition.

Vesico-ureteric reflux

Some infants suffer from a maldevelopment of the ureteric orifices leading into the bladder. Every time the bladder contracts as the patient passes urine, urine flows back into the ureters and kidney causing disease and infection. The condition may rectify itself as the structures grow larger, alternatively re-implantation of ureters has to be carried out.

Urethral valves

Urethral valves occur only in boys. They may obstruct the urinary outflow and eventually cause renal failure. The bladder becomes distended and in babies this may cause a grossly enlarged abdomen. There is a constant trickle of urine so that the napkins are wet all the time. This may lead to the condition being missed for some time. The baby may, however, be observed to strain on passing urine and later there is enuresis both day and night. A catheter can be passed quite easily as the valves merely act as an obstruction to the outflow. Urinary tract infections are common as the bladder cannot empty adequately.

The presence of valves can best be demonstrated by carrying out a voiding urethrogram. A catheter is passed into the bladder and a radio-opaque substance run in. After removing the catheter radiographs are taken while the patient voids urine and dye and empties the bladder.

In some cases the urethra can be sufficiently dilated to relieve the obstruction, but often the valves have to be excised via a perineal urethrostomy using diathermy. The prognosis depends on the amount of renal damage caused through infection and back pressure.

Neuromuscular incoordination of bladder and bladder neck

Neuromuscular incoordination causes incontinence, back pressure of urine and eventually hydronephrosis. If the hydronephrosis is bilateral, it may be necessary to transplant the ureters into a resected loop of ileum opening on to the abdominal wall. A well-fitting appliance is made to fit over the stoma and urine is collected into a bag. The mother and child must be taught to keep the stoma clean and dry. The surrounding skin needs protection by painting it with tincture of benzoin. The bag should be emptied every 4 hours and the appliance renewed as necessary and at least once a week. If disposable bags are not worn, the bag should be washed in soapy water in order to eliminate odour. The mother is given several bags to use and told to report to the hospital if the urine becomes scanty or offensive, of it the child seems off colour or is vomiting.

Ureterocele

It sometimes happens that part of the mucous lining of the bladder prolapses into it and causes obstruction of ureteric or urethral openings. This leads to stagnation of urine, back pressure, hydroureters and hydronephrosis. Treatment consists of diathermy to the prolapsed mucosa through a cystoscope or cutting and re-emplanting the ureters.

Circumcision

Surgical removal of the foreskin is done either if it is abnormally tight (phimosis), for recurrent balanitis or for religious reasons. In the neonatal period the prepuce normally adheres to the glans penis and only begins to separate after some months. Attempts to retract the foreskin routinely at bath time should therefore not be made during the first 2 or 3 years of life as forceful retraction may cause tears, infection and scarring.

Circumcision should always be carefully considered. Some authorities believe that any operation in this area should be avoided if at all possible on account of the psychological implications. Post-operatively, severe haemorrhage occurs easily and irritation of the glans, ulceration of the urethral opening from friction, ammoniacal dermatitis and meatal ulcers causing scarring and stricture are complications which result fairly frequently.

The child is admitted to hospital as a day patient and discharged towards evening. The mother is instructed to call her own doctor or bring the child back to hospital in the event of bleeding or if the child fails to pass urine. She should also be given clear instructions regarding hygiene of the area.

Post-operatively the wound edges are often covered with ribbon gauze soaked in compound tincture of benzoin and left in place for approximately 1 week. After that time it is soaked off in a bath and routine washing and dusting with some antiseptic powder are all that are required. Very occasionally the ribbon gauze has been put on too tightly and congestion and oedema of the glans result. This requires urgent relief by sitting the patient in a warm bath of potassium permanganate (two crystals to each half litre of water) and peeling the dressing off gently. Failure to do this may result in gangrene. Some surgeons leave the penis uncovered but spray the wound with Nobecutane, allowing the child to have a bath as usual from the second day. Others apply antibiotic ointment or powder instead.

During the immediate post-operative period these children are often very restless and miserable and a sedative should be given. The mother or a nurse should be available to pick the baby up and comfort him as much as possible. In uncomplicated cases there is no difficulty of micturition but the first time the child passes urine should always be noted.

Paraphimosis

Occasionally children are brought to hospital with a grossly swollen or discoloured penis caused by a tight foreskin which has been retracted but could not be returned to its normal position. Relief is a matter of urgency as the blood supply is partly cut off. Cold packs or a bath may make it possible to reduce the condition and circumcision may be undertaken at a later date. Alternatively immediate operation may be necessary if other methods fail. The skin is divided and the constriction relieved. A watch should be kept for retention of urine.

Hypospadias

Malformation of the penis and urethra may cause the urethral opening to be somewhere on the undersurface of the penis and in extreme cases it may be at the juncture of penis and scrotum. Plastic surgery aims at straightening the penis and making a new urethra from flaps of skin. The operation is usually done in two or three stages and not started until the child is about 18 months old, although meatotomy may have to be performed sooner to enlarge the urethral opening. Oedema following operation may be severe and for that reason an incision is sometimes made on the dorsum of the penis to prevent constrictive swelling and the formation of a haematoma, by allowing for adequate drainage.

The stitches are as a rule left exposed and are kept dry by dusting with an antiseptic powder. Some surgeons secure the sutures with glass beads. During the second stage, when the urethra is newly constructed, the site of operation is kept dry by the use of an in-dwelling catheter which is passed into the bladder through the perineum immediately behind the scrotum. The catheter and tubing, leading to the underwater drain containing a mild antiseptic solution, should be watched for any kinking and drainage has to be carefully measured morning and evening.

After 8–10 days the patient is allowed to pass urine through the urethra while the catheter is still in position, but spigoted and as soon as he can do so satisfactorily the in-dwelling catheter is removed. The perineal wound heals without suturing.

Following any operation on the penis or urethra, the urinal used by the patient should be sterile until the wound is healed.

All operations on the penis are extremely painful and distressing and every effort should be made to alleviate apprehension and discomfort. Sedatives should be given generously, penis and scrotum carefully supported by small pillows, the weight of the bedclothes taken by a cradle and great care taken not to pull at the catheter during bedmaking. Pressure areas need careful attention and the bowels should be watched as constipation is common and causes additional discomfort.

Undescended testicle

The testes undergo migration in fetal life from a position high up in the abdomen through the inguinal canal and into the scrotal sac. They usually reach this final position by the time of birth. In some cases, however, migration is incomplete on one or both sides. On examination it is usually possible to determine the exact position of the testicle and the length of the spermatic cord. In many cases the testicle is retractile, that is to say it lies subcutaneously near the opening of the inguinal canal and can be brought down without difficulty. Although it may retract again it can be expected to descend by the time puberty has been reached. In other cases it is ectopic and has to be brought down by operation and stitched into the scrotal sac. This is usually done at the age of 6–8 years and always before the onset of puberty. Unfortunately the testicle may be malformed and atrophic. In these cases it is removed as there is a danger of malignancy if this is not done. There may be an associated hernia, which can be repaired at the same time.

Post-operatively a few days' rest is necessary but other nursing care presents no problems. If bilateral and if left untreated, undescended testes cause sterility and in later life malignant changes may develop. Sometimes hormone therapy replaces operation but not all cases are suitable for this method of treatment and some authorities consider it to be altogether undesirable.

Exomphalos with or without ectopia vesicae

If the anterior abdominal wall is absent or if fusion of the abdominal muscles is incomplete, the abdominal and pelvic organs may be only thinly covered by amnion or peritoneum or even lie on the surface at the time of birth. The pubic bones are separated and the hip joints are abnormal. Malformation of this kind may be associated with malformations of the penis or the vagina and with absence of the urethra or bladder wall or eversion of the bladder. If this is the case, the ureteric openings can be plainly seen and there is a constant trickle of urine. Ammonia dermatitis and excoriation of the surrounding skin develop and may lead to an ascending infection of the renal tract. Until operation can be undertaken (usually at 6–12 months of age) the skin should be protected by sterile ointments and barrier creams. Moist, sterile pads are applied to absorb the urine. These should be changed at frequent intervals. Alternatively Mercurochrome solution 2% is applied. This may prevent infection and stimulate the formation of an epithelial cover.

After performing an osteotomy to approximate the pubic bones it is usually possible to suture the skin and bladder wall but it is often necessary to leave the repair of muscle to a later date. If there is a normally functioning urethra, repair is comparatively successful but often urethra and sphincter control are defective or absent and transplantation of the ureters into the sigmoid colon, ileum or rectum is necessary. The abnormal bladder is then removed at the same time. Alternatively the surgeon may divert the urine through a loop of bowel isolated from the ileum and brought on to the abdominal surface. A stick-on ileostomy bag catches the urine. It can be emptied or changed as required.

Hydrocele

A hydrocele is a swelling of the scrotum caused by fluid

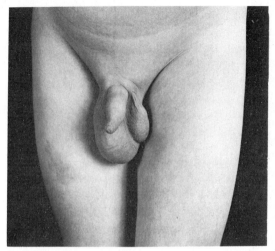

Fig. 53. A child with right hydrocele.

which accumulates in the scrotal sac. It may be unilateral or bilateral. The hydrocele may close spontaneously in the first year of life. Because of this, operation is usually delayed unless the swelling causes discomfort or embarrassment. Aspiration of the fluid is obviously useless. If operation becomes necessary, the sac is incised and the opening closed by tying off the remnant of the processus vaginalis which is present and emptying the sac.

The operation is a simple one which causes little discomfort and few problems in the after care. The child may be treated as an outpatient or as a day case (Fig. 53).

Transplantation of ureters

The operation of transplantation of ureters may have to be considered in cases in which there is either an abnormal or diseased bladder or an absence of sphincter control. This is frequently associated with malformation of the vagina, such as rectovaginal fistula.

The operation is a difficult one and as a result is often disappointing. For this reason it is more usual to create an ileal loop bladder.

The ureters are brought out on to the abdominal wall and each allowed to drain into a collecting bag.

Alternatively a loop of ileum is cut off from the alimentary canal and utilized as a reservoir, an opening made on to the surface and urine drained into a colostomy bag. This method lessens the risk of infection.

Nephrostomy

Drainage of the pelvis of the kidney is called nephrostomy. It is performed when some obstruction in the urinary tract has caused long-standing back pressure and dilatation of the ureters and renal pelvis (hydro-ureter and hydro-nephrosis) or when oedema following operation on the ureters obstructs the normal urinary flow. A Malecot catheter with a rigid tail to splint the suture line is introduced into the pelvis of the kidney and stitched in position, while a piece of corrugated rubber serves to drain the tissues around the kidney. The nephrostomy tube is kept in situ until all urinary leakage has stopped and the ureters regain their normal function. The skin around the wound should be carefully cleansed and protected against excoriation by the application of a barrier cream. Extra lengths of drainage tube are often used to allow for free movement without pulling on the tube, when this kind of drainage is used in children.

Nephrectomy

The removal of a kidney is never considered unless full investigations have shown that the other kidney is healthy and capable of taking over the total renal function. The tests carried out include intravenous pyelography, retrograde pyelography and excretion tests. It is also usual to ensure that the remaining kidney will not be at risk from the presence of infection elsewhere in the body.

Reasons for undertaking nephrectomy include congenital abnormalities of the ureters or kidney, hydronephrosis and Wilms' tumour. Tuberculosis of the kidney is rare in childhood. The child is usually admitted several days prior to operation to allow him to get used to the ward. Fluid intake and output are carefully measured for comparison with the post-operative fluid balance. In the case of Wilms' tumour, operation may be considered urgent and no time may be allowed for any special preparation unless a course of radiotherapy is given initially.

Wilms' tumour (nephroblastoma)

Wilms' tumour, which arises from the kidney, is the most commonly occurring malignant growth of childhood.

Signs and symptoms

Frequently the first signs noticed are an enlargement of the abdomen. Pain, haematuria and suppression of urine together with general malaise, anaemia and failure to thrive occur rather later and these children do in fact remain surprisingly well for a long time despite the great malignancy of the condition and its tendency to form metastases in other parts of the body, particularly the lungs. The tumour is as a rule unilateral.

Treatment

This should be started without delay. A minimum of palpation for diagnostic purposes is allowed as there is a danger of dispersing the tumour cells into the renal vein and so encouraging spread. An intravenous pyelogram will reveal distortion of the renal pelvis and displacement of the kidney. A radiograph of the chest should be taken to ensure that there is no secondary spread of the tumour to the lungs.

Operation is performed as soon as possible, blood transfusion is usually required during operation. Radiotherapy combined with cytotoxic drugs is ordered post-operatively, once the wound is healed, reducing the risk of metastases.

Further reading

BLANDY, J. (1982) *Lecture Notes on Urology*, 3rd edn. Oxford: Blackwell Scientific.

CAMERON, S. (1981) *Kidney Disease*. Oxford: Oxford University Press.

INNES-WILLIAMS, D. & JOHNSON, J. H. (1982) *Paediatric Urology*, 2nd edn. London: Butterworth.

KELALIS, P. P. & KING, L. R. (1976) *Clinical Paediatric Urology*, Vols 1 & 2. London: W. B. Saunders.

MORGAN, R. (1981) *Childhood Incontinence*. London: Heinemann Medical.

16 Infection and communicable diseases

SCABIES *(Sarcoptes scabiei)*

Scabies is a skin infection caused by a minute parasite. The female mite burrows into the skin, most commonly between the fingers, and lays her eggs; it is usually possible to see the burrows with the help of a magnifying glass. As the eggs hatch, the larvae move to the hair follicles. Intense irritation results and this is particularly marked when the skin becomes warm at night. In young babies the soft skin allows for access in any part of the body and lesions can be found anywhere. In those babies who have not started walking, lesions may even occur on the soft skin of the soles of the feet. Secondary infections are common as a result of scratching. The infection occurs as a result of direct contact with an infected person or through indirect contact with soiled bed linen, clothing, etc.

Treatment

The child is given a warm bath which softens the skin and opens the burrows to allow penetration of the prescribed lotion; the skin is then dry. The lotion is applied—benzyl benzoate or gamma benzene hexachloride—taking care to work in between the toes, fingers and other flexures. After 24 hours the whole procedure is repeated.

All clothing, underwear and bed linen should be changed. All members of the family should be treated at the same time.

It is not necessary to send blankets or other garments for disinfection but all clothing, underwear and bed linen should be laundered.

It is important to tell the parents that the lesions may persist for several months despite successful treatment, irritation too may continue. Calamine may be applied to ease this irritation.

HEAD LICE (Pediculosis capitis)

The incidence of infestation with head lice continues to rise each year, school children being the most commonly infested. Infestation of the hair by head lice should be suspected if the child is noticed to be scratching the scalp frequently, particularly at the back, as the head lice tend to inhabit the occipital region rather than the front part of the scalp. Secondary infection of the scratches on the scalp may produce a coincident impetigo. In some children, where infestation is severe, cervical adenitis associated with malaise and pyrexia may occur as a result of secondary infection.

The louse reproduces by means of hatching eggs which are attached to hair follicles close to the scalp by means of a 'cement-like' substance. This makes the removal of the eggs or 'nits' difficult.

Treatment

The basis of successful treatment is both educational and practical. It is essential that the whole family be treated and this should include all the adults as well as any pre-school children.

Pediculosis capitis may be treated with Malathion or Carbaryl according to the manufacturers' instructions. Twelve hours after the use of either preparation, the hair is shampooed and combed with a fine comb whilst still wet. It is not necessary after treatment to comb out the 'nits' or eggs, which can be uncomfortable for the child. These eggs die and any eggs found more than half an inch away from the scalp are harmless.

CATSCRATCH FEVER

Probably a virus infection. Cat apparently healthy. A few days after scratch, ulcer or sore. A week or two later—regional lymph nodes very enlarged, some fever. Nodes may suppurate or adenitis persist for some months. Pus sterile, white cell count normal. Treated with broad-spectrum antibiotic to prevent suppuration.

TOXOCARIASIS (Visceral larva migrans)

Toxocariasis is an infection caused by the transmission of the visceral larvae migrans. These are deposited in the soil from dog and cat faeces. Children 1–4 years of age are the most likely to be infected, especially if they have a 'dirt-eating habit'. When the ova are swallowed, the larvae hatch in the intestine, pass through the intestinal wall and wander through the viscera. They pass first to the liver and then to other intestinal organs, where they may produce granulomas. These are most commonly found in the liver but can also occur in the kidney, heart, striated muscle, brain and eyeball. Common presenting symptoms are fever, skin rash with general malaise and anorexia. As the larvae migrate, haemorrhage, granuloma formation and chest infections with enlarged tender liver and spleen occur. Ophthalmitis may occur in severe infections. There is an associated eosinophilia. Diagnosis is difficult although a standardized skin test is available. With many children a spontaneous improvement is common. Treatment is symptomatic.

Prevention is the most effective weapon against this infection. All pet dogs and cats should be given regular periodic anthelmintics. Dogs should not be allowed to foul children's playing areas or foot paths.

INTESTINAL PARASITES

Threadworms (Pinworms—*Enterobius vermicularis*)

Threadworm infestation is exceedingly common in children, and entire families may be affected.

The threadworm normally inhabits the large intestine but the female migrates to the anal region where she deposits her eggs. Irritation, particularly during the night, causes the child to scratch and reinfect himself through his finger nails. Sharing beds and towels is an obvious way in which infection is spread to others.

Signs and symptoms

The most general symptom is itching and this in turn may cause restless sleep and irritability. Scratching and irritation may cause inflammation of the perineum, vulvovaginitis, bed-wetting and occasionally diarrhoea or rectal prolapse.

The tiny worms may first be noticed in the course of a toilet round, although the worms remain on the surface of the stool only momentarily and then disappear into its substance. Alternatively the mother may describe symptoms which suggest the diagnosis.

Diagnostic test

In order to prove the presence of threadworms a simple test can be done. A piece of Sellotape 2.5 cm (1 in.) wide and 7.6 cm (3 in.) long is placed, sticky side down, on the perineum immediately on waking. It is then transferred to a microscope slide, again sticky side down and labelled and sent to the laboratory. The threadworm ova are obvious under the microscope. As the procedure is such a simple one it can easily be carried out by an outpatient's mother.

Treatment

Careful hygiene is the first essential. Finger nails should be kept short and hand washing before meals should be enforced. Pyjamas should be worn in preference to night gowns and both pyjamas and day knickers should be washed and boiled daily. At night cotton mittens can be worn to prevent infecting the finger nails. The local application of an analgesic ointment is useful to relieve rectal irritation.

Drug therapy

Piperazine hydrate (0.25–2 g twice daily for 7 days) may be given. Pripsen, a granular compound containing piperazine phosphate and standardized senna, as Senokot. It is effective when given in one single dose. However, in order to exclude possible reinfestation during the first 2 days after treatment, when occasional ova may still be present, a second dose is often given after a week or 10 days. Vanquin, another single dose anthelmintic, is equally effective. All members of the family should be treated.

RINGWORM

A fungus infection caused by a microsporon is responsible for this skin condition. Ringworm usually affects the scalp or nails of school children and is highly contagious.

Since the advent of the oral antibiotic drug griseofulvin, the former routine treatment with X-rays has been abandoned. The diagnosis is confirmed by examination under a Wood's glass filter which shows the hair with a characteristic fluorescent green colour.

ATHLETE'S FOOT (Tinea interdigitalis)

This very common condition, due to an epidermophyton, is highly contagious. The disease is spread through towels, bath mats and communal baths, becoming a particular problem in boarding schools. Areas of sodden skin with cracks and fissures appear between the toes, spreading to the sole of the foot which may become quite sore.

Treatment

The sodden skin should be removed each day and zinc undecylenate ointment applied. This substance is also available as a dusting powder to be used in socks and shoes. Treatment should be continued for at least a week after the last sign of infection has disappeared to prevent a relapse. Meticulous attention to hygiene is essential to prevent the spread of this infection to others. Where a pupil is reported with this condition attention must be paid by the authorities to the bathroom and swimming pool floors to avoid an outbreak throughout the school.

GASTROENTERITIS

Gastroenteritis should always be considered as a potentially serious condition. Mild symptoms may quickly develop into a more serious disease. It occurs in almost any age group. Pre-term babies are particularly prone to gastroenteritis, but it is rarely seen in breast-fed babies.

The infection is as a rule due to various strains of *Escherichia* (*Bacterium*) *coli*, salmonella or dysentery bacillus, and possibly to some as yet unidentified virus. Other types are secondary to infection outside the gastrointestinal tract such as middle ear infections, meningitis or the common cold. Symptoms similar to those caused by infective gastroenteritis may be due to dietetic errors and disaccharide intolerance.

Nursing management

Strict precautions against spread of infection must be observed. Where other infants are nursed in the same unit, ideally no nurse attending a case of infective gastroenteritis should handle these or be allowed into the feed kitchen (see p. 28).

The symptoms of gastroenteritis in infancy may vary from slight frequency of the bowel actions, relaxed stools and an occasional vomit, to a severe illness with gross dehydration and generalized disturbances. For the purpose of this chapter a severe, fully established case is described.

The mother will explain that the infant has had increasingly frequent, loose and explosive stools with a characteristic, offensive smell and that his buttocks are becoming sore. She may have noticed traces of blood or mucus in the stools, or she may have seen bits of curd and free fluid. The colour may be green or bright orange. An observant mother may even have noticed that her baby is passing very little and rather dark urine, a sure sign of severe dehydration and incipient renal failure. She will say that the baby is wakeful, restless and constantly whimpering. Although he appears to be thirsty and to want his feeds, he is often unable to retain them and the vomiting may be forceful and copious and occur during or immediately after taking a feed. Vomiting, however, is not a constant feature. As he gets worse, the baby may refuse his feeds. It is obvious that loss of weight will be rapid and severe, and that all the signs of dehydration and loss of electrolytes will soon be present.

The loss of 150–300 ml will cause a baby to look very ill. Particular attention must be paid to the sodium level in the blood which becomes high during dehydration. Deep, rapid respirations are characteristic of acidosis, and an increase in the vomiting, spasms and convulsions are often signs of severe alkalosis.

Blood is taken for biochemical analysis and any electrolyte imbalance is corrected without delay. In vomiting, chlorides are lost to the body and diarrhoea causes loss of sodium and potassium. These deficiencies must be made good by giving intravenous fluids urgently, as young infants deteriorate very rapidly. It is often necessary to start treatment without waiting for the result of laboratory tests.

A specimen of stool should be sent to the laboratory, while fresh. If a rectal swab is taken it may be moistened by dipping it in sterile broth solution, as used for blood cultures, before insertion into the rectum.

Special observations

It is important that any complication should be noticed early because no time should be lost before appropriate treatment is started. Any change in the infant must be reported without delay and its significance understood.

Bearing in mind the symptoms of the disease and the complications already mentioned, the nurse will closely observe the following points.

1. The condition of the skin; hot or cold, dry or clammy, pale, flushed, inelastic or jaundiced.

2. The fontanelles; sunken or bulging.

3. The mouth; dryness, the lips cracked or the tongue red or coated. Look for signs of thrush (see p. 202).

4. The baby's attitude; restlessness or lethargy. Do the eyes look sunken?

5. Note any excoriation of the buttocks and any swelling of the abdomen.

6. Record any urine passed; the amount and colour. If possible save a specimen for testing for any abnormalities.

7. Observe any stool for mucus, free fluid and blood.

Rectal temperatures should never be taken, as the irritation of introducing the thermometer into the rectum may cause unnecessary bowel actions. It is always necessary to correlate these observations and to judge the condition of the patient as a whole, when deciding on treatment and diet, instead of noting only the number and frequency of the stools.

Feeding

Once the electrolyte and serum protein losses have been corrected by intravenous therapy, oral feeding can be started and it is rarely necessary to continue with intravenous fluids for longer than 36 hours.

The first feeds offered should be boiled water and glucose 4.3% or dextrose in 1/5 normal saline solution. (A suitable mixture may be made by using one tablespoon of sugar to 1/4 teaspoon of salt in 1 pint (0.6 litres) of boiled water.) Extra fluid, 300 ml daily to make up for loss of fluid. Milk in dilution is gradually introduced until the infant's usual feed has been re-established. Expressed breast milk may be invaluable in some cases.

Table 9. Table of communicable diseases

Disease	Incubation period	Organism and mode of spread	Signs and symptoms	Treatment and complications	Other remarks
Mumps	14–28 days	Virus Droplet	Fever, malaise, stiff jaw, swelling of salivary gland—parotid and submandibular. Unilateral or bilateral. Trismus. Pain on eating—especially sugars. Furred tongue, mouth dry—diminution of saliva. Moderate lymphocytosis.	Symptomatic. Mouth care—drink with straw. Avoid foods which are sweet and stimulate salivary glands. Mastitis, oophoritis, prostatitis, pancreatitis (all rare), meningitis, encephalitis (may lead to permanent deafness), facial paralysis. Orchitis at or after puberty.	Complement fixation test reaction to confirm diagnosis—rarely necessary.
Glandular fever (infectious mononucleosis)	6–14 days	*Epstein-Barr virus (EBV)* Droplet. Low infectivity.	Lassitude, anorexia, general malaise, pyrexia, headache, sore throat with tonsillar exudate which separates easily without bleeding. May be petechiae on palate. Enlarged lymph nodes and spleen. Transient macular rash—chest trunk, limbs and particularly dorsum of hands and feet. Leucocytosis with raised monocytes (atypical). Paul Bunnell test may be positive.	Symptomatic. Treat general debility and depression—prolonged convalescence. Treat secondary infections—hepatitis, meningitis, encephalitis. Nephritis.	Relapses common, but complete recovery eventually.
Diphtheria	2–7 days	*Corynebacterium diphtheriae*	Malaise, headache, rapid, feeble pulse, some rise in temperature, toxic. Albuminuria, exhaustion.	Diphtheria antitoxin if any question of infection possible. Absolute bed rest, mouth care, tube feed if necessary.	Notifiable. Follow up contacts and possible carriers. Treat carriers with antibiotic and possibly tonsil-

Disease	Incubation	Spread	Clinical features	Complications	Treatment	Prevention/Control
		Droplet	*Faucial:* Slight sore throat, continuous greyish membrane spreading to soft palate and pharynx, which bleeds when attempt made to remove. Glands of neck very enlarged. 'Bull neck'. myocarditis. *Nasal:* Thin bloodstained nasal discharge with offensive smell. Crusting of external nares. *Laryngeal:* Croupy cough, laryngeal stridor, loss of voice, asphyxia.	Myocarditis, paralysis of limbs, palate, diaphragm, ciliary muscles and external rectus muscles, nephritis, peripheral neuritis.	Tracheotomy may become necessary. Penicillin to treat secondary infection. Mechanical ventilation will be necessary if diaphragm paralysed. Physiotherapy after acute stage.	Immunization advisable to prevent infection and epidemics. Schick test to assess immunity—negative if immune.
Enteric fever	2 weeks	Typhoid (*Salmonella typhi*). Paratyphoid A, B and 'C' (*S. paratyphi* A, B and C) (non-lactose fermenters). Contamination of food or water by excreta from carriers or patients with the disease. Fomites, flies	Headache, tiredness, aching limbs, cough, fever rising in 'step-ladder' fashion, relative bradycardia, palpable spleen, abdominal discomfort, 'rose spots' on abdomen or chest—constipated—later 'pea soup' stools. Leucopenia if no secondary infection. Typhoid state—drowsy, confused, muttering, plucking at bedclothes, 'coma vigil'. Blood culture positive in first few days. Widal test—rising titre.	Venous thrombosis, acute arthritis, cholecystitis, bone abscess and periostitis, peritonitis. Parotitis if inadequate mouth care.	Symptomatic. High calorie, low roughage, diet. Care of mouth and skin. Watch for haemorrhage from perforated Peyer's patches. Transfusion if necessary.	Notifiable. Isolate until 2 negative stool cultures (consecutive). Immunize contacts. Treat carriers—if necessary with cholecystectomy.

Table 9. Table of communicable diseases—contd.

Disease	Incubation period	Organism and mode of spread	Signs and symptoms	Treatment and complications	Other remarks
Brucellosis (undulant fever)	1–3 weeks	*Brucella abortus* (cattle) *Brucella melitensis* (goats). *Brucella suis* (pigs). Infected, unpasteurized milk, meat, dairy products. Infected hides and carcases.	Headache, malaise, anorexia, constipation, fever—settles by lysis in 10 days, but recurs. Cough, backache, profuse sweating, palpable spleen. Transient arthritis. *Abortus fever* (chronic brucellosis). Insidious, milder and more prolonged. Recurrent night sweats without serious general ill health. (*In both*) Blood culture may be positive. Rising agglutination titre. Leucopenia, mild anaemia.	Tetracycline streptomycin, vitamin B. Symptomatic—treat debility with long convalescence. Disinfect excreta—especially urine.	Notifiable. Recurring at short intevals for many months. Pasteurization of milk, clean water and destroying infected animals prevents disease.
Roseola infantum (exanthema subitum, sixth disease, pseudorubella)	8–15 days	Virus Droplets	Fever, macular rash—appears immediately temperature fallen, fades on pressure. On trunk, neck, proximal part of limbs; *not* face. Lasts 1–3 days. Little malaise. Catarrhal pharyngitis, cervical lymphadenopathy. Neutrophil leucopenia with relative lymphocytosis.	Symptomatic. Convulsions due to high fever.	Practically confined to first 3 years of life.

Disease	Incubation	Organism	Spread	Signs and symptoms	Treatment	Complications	Notes
Measles (morbilli)	10–14 days	Virus	Droplet	Running eyes and nose. Dry, irritating cough. Conjunctivitis. Photophobia. Pyrexia. Transient prodromal rash. Koplik spots—white on red base on buccal mucous membrane. 3rd day: temperature subsides. 4th day: rash appears—dusky red macular rash behind ears → face, trunk, limbs. Temperature again elevated. Rash becomes large irregular blotchy areas of darker red.	Bed. Symptomatic. Antibiotic for secondary infections.	Otitis media. Blepharitis. Corneal ulcerations. Bronchopneumonia. Collapsed lobe of lung. Bronchiectasis and lung abscess (if collapse insufficiently treated). Tuberculosis. Encephalitis and encephalomyelitis (gastroenteritis in infancy.)	Notifiable. Segregate until rash fades. Passive immunity for 3 months after birth (if mother has had measles). Older or sick children are given convalescent serum 5–10 ml or adult serum or gamma-globulin for protection. *Gamma globulin* 250 mg prevent attack under 1 year, attenuates attack at all ages. Later 750 mg should prevent attack. Second dose after 6 weeks.
German measles (rubella)	14–21 days	Virus	Droplet	Mild malaise and pyrexia day before rash. Generalized tender lymphadenitis especially posterior cervical and occipital. Rash: pink macules and papules at first discrete then confluent.	Very little necessary—symptomatic.	Occasionally: Encephalitis. Arthritis.	Danger to fetus during first 14 weeks in utero if mother affected. Baby may be born deaf, with cataract, glaucoma, or heart disease (also risk of abortion). Mother should be given gamma globulin.
Scarlet fever (scarlatina)	1–7 days	Haemolytic streptococci (Lancefield Group A)	Droplet, fomites, milk	Headache, vomiting, pyrexia. Sore throat—soft yellow exudate. 'Strawberry tongue'. Polymorphonuclear leucocytosis. Raised antistreptolysin titre. Cervical lymphadenitis. Rash—punctuate erythema, bright scarlet, behind ears and sides of neck → whole body except circumoral pallor. Desquamation after 1 week.	(Septic and toxic forms very rare.) Bed. Penicillin and sulphonamides. Fluids. Mouth care.	Pneumonia. Septicaemia. Otitis media. Acute nephritis and rheumatism. Anaphylactoid purpura. Sinusitis. Encephalitis. Quinsy. Retropharyngeal abscess. Cervical adenitis and abscess.	Notifiable. Dick test for diagnosis—rarely used. Possibility of cardiac lesions from acute rheumatism. Scarlet fever antitoxin sometimes given.

Table 9. Table of communicable diseases—contd.

Disease	Incubation period	Organism and mode of spread	Signs and symptoms	Treatment and complications	Other remarks
Whooping cough (pertussis)	7–14 days	*Bordetella* (*Haemophilus*) *pertussis* Droplet	Cold → chest infection → cough which becomes paroxysmal with vomiting and may end with a whoop. Ulcer on fraenum. Lymphocytosis. Low erythrocyte sedimentation rate. Baby vomits, cyanosed, limp, no paroxysms.	Feed after vomiting. Sedation. Broad-spectrum antibiotics for secondary infections. Deal with debility—long convalescence, high-calorie diet. Otitis media. Bronchopneumonia. Pulmonary collapse. Bronchiectasis. Tuberculosis. Subconjunctival haemorrhage. Cerebral anoxia or haemorrhage. Convulsions. Hernia. Rectal prolapse. Spontaneous pneumothorax.	Notifiable. No passive immunity in babies. Mild abortive case in immunized child, but equally infectious. Child often 'whoops' for months after attack—not infectious. Routine immunization—not to child with epilepsy or prone to convulsions—he may develop encephalopathy if immunized. Resuscitation equipment and oxygen available in case a severe apnoeic attack should occur.

N.B. For the infant under 3 months the best protection against whooping cough is the vaccination of all siblings.

Disease	Incubation period	Organism and mode of spread	Signs and symptoms	Treatment and complications	Other remarks
Chickenpox (varicella)	14–21 days	Virus Contact and droplet	Minimal malaise and headache. Fever. Transient prodromal rash. Main rash appears in crops—mainly on face, head and trunk (centripetal) oval, unilocular papules → vesicles → pustules → crusts. Irritating rash. Lymphocytosis.	Prevent from scratching to avoid scarring. Baths. Calamine. Keep cool. Short nails. Elbow splints if necessary. Antihistamines. Antibiotics for secondary infections—impetigo, boils, cellulitis, conjunctivitis, polyneuritis, encephalitis, transverse myelitis.	Herpes zoster closely allied. Severe or fatal if child has leukaemia or is on steroid therapy. Segregate until scabs dry.

Disease	Incubation period	Cause/Transmission	Signs and symptoms	Nursing care/Treatment	Prevention
Poliomyelitis	5–21 days	Virus, through gastro-intestinal tract.	Sore throat, headache, stiff neck. Muscle weakness.	Bed rest. Symptomatic treatment. Paralysis.	Vaccination available (see p. 19).
Tuberculosis	3–12 weeks	Mycobacterium tuberculosis. Close contact with infected person. Droplet.	The majority of children show little clinical upset. Vague and non-specific. Fever, loss of appetite and weight, lassitude and headache. However, specific symptoms will vary according to system attacked.	Nursing care aimed at symptomatic relief. Long-term chemotherapy with antituberculous drugs.	Prophylaxis with BCG (see p. 20).
Tetanus	3 days to 3 weeks	Clostridium tetani found in soil. Through break in skin.	Fever, feels unwell. Stiffening of jaw. 1–2 days later spastic rigidity of the body.	Bed rest in quiet dark room. Reduce muscle spasms, maintain hydration. Clean wound. Convulsions leading to death.	Tetanus immunoglobulin or antitoxin.
Infective hepatitis	15–40 days	Virus: type A; type B. Contaminated food. Faecal/oral route. Infected blood products.	Fever, headache, anorexia, nausea, abdominal pain, myalgias.	Bed rest initially. Disinfect excreta. Offer frequent fluids with added glucose. Light nutritious diet. Slow recovery. N.B. Use disposable syringes and needles. Dispose of carefully according to unit policy.	

ISOLATION NURSING MANAGEMENT

The aim of care is to prevent the spread of infection from the infected child to another using barrier nursing techniques. For other children who are susceptible to infection, e.g. those with immunosuppressive problems, the aim is to protect the child using reverse barrier nursing techniques. Specific nursing procedures vary from unit to unit but the following principles will apply.

Accommodation

Ideally nursing care should take place in a cubicle with its own hand basin, soap and hand towel dispenser, where the child can be observed easily through glass panes. All equipment and furniture in the cubicle should be easy to clean and maintain. The doors to the cubicle should preferably be of the swing type so that entering and leaving can be made easily without contamination of the hands.

Equipment in cubicle

1. Bins and plastic bin-liners with good seals, for soiled hand towels, linen and disposables.
2. Basic items for physical examination, e.g. spatula, tape-measure, stethoscope, etc.
3. Small amount of clean linen.
4. Cleaning equipment.

Nursing records and charts are best left outside the cubicle except for those charts needed for immediate recording of frequent observations.

Gowns

Gowns should be worn if the child, bed, bedding or clothing is handled. Two gowns should be provided which will need changing daily. When worn, these should be put on and taken off correctly (see p. 28).

Tapes should always be tied at the neck and waist. Unless a clean gown is used each time, the outside of the gown should always be considered contaminated.

Masks

Paper masks should only be worn for 15–20 minutes in the following circumstances:

1. In the case of a child with an acute infectious disease.
2. In circumstances where the child is at great risk of acquiring infection, i.e. the child with a low white blood cell count.

Incorrectly used masks do more harm than good and the handling of masks under any circumstances is to be avoided once they are in use.

Hand washing technique

Careful hand washing technique by all members of the staff before touching a child who is being nursed with an isolation nursing technique. This has been shown to be the single most important factor in reducing the spread of infection. Hands should be washed and dried well, before and after wearing a protective gown.

Parents and other visitors will need careful instruction and supervision in hand washing techniques, and in the wearing of gowns and masks.

Cleaning

Particular attention should be paid to the cleaning of all hand basins and water outlets and all other services. These should be cleaned by a member of the domestic staff who has been carefully instructed in the technique to be followed.

Disposal of Excreta

1. Infants should wear disposal nappies which can be sealed in the appropriate bag and disposed of.

2. Usually excreta in bed pans/potties can be disposed of using the bed pan sterilizer in the normal way. However, if the infection is due to typhoid or polio the faeces should be soaked, e.g. with an appropriate disinfectant, for one hour. The bed pan is then disinfected and cleaned in the usual way.

Disposal of foods and feeds

Wherever possible disposable utensils should be used. Left over scraps of food can be disposed of in the appropriate bin. Left over milk feeds or fluids can be disposed of down the sink.

Terminal disinfection after the discharge of known infectious cases

1. Blankets, linen, clothing, etc. should be sent in sealed plastic bags to the foul washer in the laundry.

2. All disposable equipment should be incinerated.

3. Soft toys should be placed in bags, and sterilized if possible or burnt in the incinerator.

4. Furniture, walls and floors should be washed with soap and water and the room left to air thoroughly for several hours.

N.B. In some circumstances the cubicle may be sealed and disinfected with formaldehyde gas. This is usually carried out by the hospital works department and is usually ordered when the infection has been due to a particularly virulent organism.

Further reading

CHRISTIE, A. B. (1980) *Infectious Diseases*. London: Churchill Livingstone.

DICK, G. (1978) *Immunisation*. London: Update Books.

Department of Health and Social Security (1982) *Immunisation Against Infectious Disease*, Revised Memoranda. London: DHSS.

Department of Health and Social Security (1981) *Whooping Cough.* Report from the Committee on Safety of Medicine and the Joint Committee on Vaccination and Immunisation. London: HMSO.

ILLINGWORTH, R. S. (1981) *Infectious Immunisation of Your Child.* London: Churchill Livingstone.

MARKS, M. I. (1979) *Common Bacterial Infections of Infancy and Childhood.* Lancaster: M.T.P. Press.

Appendix 1
Safety

Prevention of accidents

Dangers	How to guard against them in home and hospital
	Fires
Electric fires, gas fires, coal fires	Efficient guards fixed to fire surround. Fix on wall whenever possible. Wire netting fixed to fire.
	Electricity
Sockets	Locked sockets prevent children from poking fingers or pointed articles into the holes. 'Baby Guards' can be obtained to fit over all 5, 13 and 15 amp British plugs.
Flexes	Short flexes prevent accidents, i.e. tripping over them. Long flexes tempt children to pull on them, e.g. flex from electric iron.
	Hot water
Water taps	Fix out of reach if possible. Never leave child alone in bathroom.
Baths	Run cold water in before the hot to prevent floor of bath from getting too hot.
Bath water	Mix well, test with elbow.
Hot-water bottles	Use tap (not boiling) water. Cover completely with two protective layers. Never give hot water bottles to unconscious or paralysed patients.
	Scalds
Teapots, kettles	Point spout away from table or stove edge. Drinking from the spouts of teapots and kettles seems attractive to the very young child. Oedema of the mouth, larynx and oesophagus may necessitate tracheostomy. Keep well out of the way.

Tablecloths	Tablecloths should not be used or should at least not exceed the size of the table surface. If allowed to hang over table edge the toddler may tug on them when wanting to reach something on the table. Serious scalds may result if there is a teapot on the table.
Saucepans	Saucepan handles should always be directed backwards or inwards. Safety rails for stoves are available. The child may reach for the handle in an attempt at 'peeping inside' to see what is cooking.
Buckets	Buckets filled with scalding water should never be left standing on the floor unguarded. The young child may fall or plunge his hands into it.

Swallowing and inhaling

Toys	Toys should be large enough to make it impossible for younger children to swallow or inhale them.
	Beads, nails and small marbles should not be given to very young toddlers.
	Toys should not have sharp edges—danger of cuts and abrasions.
	They should be coloured with vegetable (not lead) paint.

Suffocation

Pillows	Should not be used in cots before the age of 1 year or until the child can safely move himself. They are particularly dangerous if they are soft.
Plastic bibs	Avoid. They may fall over the baby's face and interfere with breathing.
Plastic bags	Children should never be allowed to play with these.

Gangrene

Mittens	These are best avoided. A thread of cotton or strand of wool hanging off the inside edge of the mitten has been known to wrap itself round the tip of a finger causing constriction and gangrene.

Foreign bodies

Small objects	All body orifices offer opportunities for young children to push beads, peas, ball of paper, etc., into them. Sepsis and foul-smelling discharge will result. The observant and watchful mother or nurse should spot the toddler doing this sort of thing before the harm is done.

Prevention of accidents—contd.

Dangers	How to guard against them in home and hospital
	Sharp things
Knives, saws, axes, scissors	All these should be kept out of harm's way. If left lying around they are likely to be misused and dangerous. Playing with them should be forbidden, while very young. When a little older their use should be supervised. The 'first' scissors should have rounded ends and they should not be too sharp. A child who has 'his own' will not want adult ones.
Safety pins	Should always be fastened when not in use. If in use they should be inaccessible to the child. On napkins they should be pinned horizontally.
Pin boxes, needle books	Should be kept well out of reach.
	Fire and burning
Matches	Children should be taught to respect matches as dangerous.
Matchboxes	Should not be left lying around the house.
Lighters	The same applies to them as to matches.
Fireworks and bonfires	Children should know that both may be enjoyed only while supervised by adults.
Clothing	Pyjamas are preferable for girls as well as boys as their closer fit diminishes the danger of catching fire.
	Flame-proofed materials are obtainable, their advantages greatly outweigh the extra cost.
Mirrors, pictures	Should not be fixed over fireplaces. Clothes easily catch fire as one leans over the fireplace to look in the mirror.
	Windows
Guards	Safety guards should be fixed on windows of any rooms in which young children may have to be left alone.
Chairs, step ladders	May invite the child to climb on to them and lean out of the window. If unguarded this may have serious results.
	Stairs
Safety gates	When there is a toddler in the house stairs should be made safe by placing safety gates at the top and bottom of flights of stairs.

Poisoning

Solvents	Young people should be aware of the health problems of 'glue sniffing'. Counselling and support groups should be provided for adolescents to discuss the hazard of solvent abuse.
Disinfectants	Should be kept locked away or out of reach even if the toddler climbs to get at them.
	They should always be clearly labelled, but it must also be remembered that the child may not be able to read. Disinfectants should not be stored in old fruit-juice bottles which still have the original label on.
Pills tablets, medicines	As the young child loves putting things in his mouth, pills, etc., should be inaccessible to him. These should be kept in a locked cupboard.
Berries	A firm warning against picking and eating berries must be given in early days.
Cosmetics	Cosmetics should be kept out of reach of toddlers as some are harmful when taken internally.

Water safety

Paddling, swimming	Young children should be taught to swim early in life. The child should be shown danger spots such as sudden drops in depth, dangerous currents and outlets from drains. When on holiday by lake, sea or river, children should wear safety belts or jackets.
	Parents should insist on children paddling or swimming where other people are about.

Road safety

Road deaths and injuries	The Safety Code should be taught untiringly by parents and in schools.

Appendix 2
Toy Libraries
Association

Toy Libraries initially catered for the needs of physically and mentally handicapped children as well as mentally handicapped adults. Today they open their doors to all children with special needs, including those in hospital, so that they may benefit from playing with, and borrowing from, a selection of carefully chosen toys. A lonely child is often an unhappy child and a Toy Library provides children with an opportunity to meet and play with other children in an exciting but caring environment.

Others too can benefit from belonging to a Toy Library. The brothers and sisters of the handicapped child are welcome. There are those with less obvious (although no less real) problems, e.g. families suffering from emotional or social stress. There are groups of people such as childminders and foster parents who seek the advice, and benefit from the help, that a Toy Library is able to offer.

A Toy Library provides good quality (and sometimes specially adapted) toys which may be borrowed and taken home to extend the children's enjoyment and therapy. It is also a meeting place where parents, volunteer helpers and professional advisers can meet informally. Problems are shared, ideas exchanged and many family friendships are made.

Many good quality toys are expensive and so parents, if they can afford to, hesitate to buy in case their child does not enjoy them. A Toy Library gives the parents and child a chance to experiment with a wide selection of toys. Then favourites can be bought with confidence.

THE AIMS OF THE ASSOCIATION

The object of the Association shall be the relief and education of all handicapped children by the provision of therapeutic, educational and stimulating toys and equipment, and in furtherance of such an object the Association shall aim to:

(a) Further the setting up of charitable independent Toy Libraries in this country, whose purpose shall be to:

396

(1) Assist the development, from the earliest age, of all handicapped children whatever their disability in the towns or areas covered by each of them.
(2) Provide the best available toys to them.
(3) Provide an opportunity for professional involvement in a voluntary service for handicapped children.

(b) Foster the understanding of play needs of handicapped children and to give guidance on the selection of good toys and play materials.

(c) Promote, work for, and maintain communication between:
(1) Individual Toy Libraries.
(2) Professional workers and Toy Libraries.
(3) Manufacturers, designers and other interested bodies and Toy Libraries societies for the Handicapped and Toy Libraries.

HOW TO LOCATE YOUR NEAREST TOY LIBRARY

Write to the Toy Libraries Association, Seabrook House, Wyllyotts Manor, Darkes Lane, Potters Bar, Hertfordshire, EN6 2HL. The Toy Libraries Association will provide you with the address of your nearest Toy Library (as it is a charity please remember to send a stamped addressed envelope). It will also give you invaluable advice on how to start a Toy Library in your own neighbourhood if the established library is inconveniently situated.

The Toy Library Association also organizes training programmes for those interested in setting up a Toy Library and will provide, on request, an initiation pack full of information and ideas about the actual mechanism of founding a local Toy Library in an area where one does not already exist. Membership of the Toy Library Association can be either as an individual, or as a Toy Library or as a commercial concern. Membership for those living overseas can also be obtained.

PUBLICATIONS

The Toy Libraries Association produces many useful booklets and other publications. Details of these are given at the end of the appropriate chapters in the further reading lists

Appendix 3
Useful addresses

Association for All Speech-Impaired Children (*AFASIC*), 347 Central Markets, Smithfield, London EC1A 9NH. (01-236 3632)

Association of British Paediatric Nurses, The Hon. Secretary, c/o Central Nursing Office, The Hospital for Sick Children, Great Ormond Street, London WC1.

Association of Parents of Vaccine-Damaged Children, 2 Church Street, Shipston-on-Stour, Warwicks, CV36 4AP.

Association for Research into Restricted Growth, 2 Mount Court, 81 Central Hill, London SE19 1BS.

Association for Spina Bifida and Hydrocephalus, Tavistock House North, Tavistock Square, London WC1H 9HJ. (01-388 1382)

British Deaf Association, 38 Victoria Place, Carlisle CA1 1HU (0228 20188). Mainly concerned with adults; some publications relevant to children.

British Diabetic Association, 3-4 Alfred Place, London WC1E 7EE. (01-636 7355)

British Epilepsy Association, 3-6 Alfred Place, London WC1E 7EE. (01–580 2704)

British Heart Foundation, 57 Gloucester Place, London W1H 4DH. (01-935 0185)

British Kidney Patient Association, Bordon, Hants. (042-03 2021)

Brittle Bone Society, 63 Byron Crescent, Dundee DD3 6SS. (0382-87130)

Chest and Heart Association, Tavistock House North, Tavistock Square, London WC1H 9HJ. (01-387 3012)

Children's Chest Circle, Tavistock House North, Tavistock Square, London WC1.

Cleft Lip and Palate Association, Dental Dept, The Hospital for Sick Children, Great Ormond Street, London WC1N 3JH. (01-405 9200)

Colostomy Welfare Group, 38 Eccleston Square, London SW1U 1PB. (01-828 5175)

Cystic Fibrosis Research Trust, 5 Blyth Road, Bromley, Kent BR1 3RS. (01-461 7211)

Down's Children's Association, Quinbourne Community Centre, Ridgacre Road, Birmingham B32 2TW. (021-427 1374)

Foundation for the Study of Infant Deaths, 23 St Peter's Square, London W6 9NW. (01-235 1721) (out of office hours 01-748 7768)

Genetic Counselling: every General Practitioner should hold a list issued by the Department of Health and Social Security.

Haemophilia Society, PO Box 9, 16 Trinity Street, London SE1 1DE. (01-407 1010)

Handicapped children, supplies and equipment:

E. J. Arnold & Son Ltd, Buttersley Street, Leeds.

James Galt & Co. Ltd, Brookfield Road, Cheadle, Cheshire.

Task Master Ltd, Morris Road, Clarendon Park, Leicester.

Lady Hoare Trust for Physically Disabled Children, 7 North Street, Midhurst, W. Sussex GU29 9 DJ. (073-081 3696)

Leukaemia Research Fund, 61 Great Ormond Street, London WC1. (01-405 9200)

Leukaemia Society, 28 Eastern Road, London N2. (01-883 4703)

Muscular Dystrophy Group of Great Britain, Nattrass House, 35 Macaulay Road, London SW4 OQP. (01-720 8055)

National Advisory Centre for Battered Children, Denver House, Bound's Green Road, London N11

National Association for Deaf/Blind and Rubella Children, 164 Cromwell Lane, Coventry CV4 8AP, Warwicks. (0203-462579)

National Association for the Education of the Partially Sighted, Joseph Clark School, Vincent Road, Higham Park, London E4. (01-527 8818)

National Association for Gifted Children, 1 South Audley Street, London W1.

National Association for Maternity and Child Welfare, 1 South Audley Street, London W1.

National Association for Mental Handicap, 5 Fitzwilliam Place, Dublin. ((Dublin) 76 6035)

National Association for the Welfare of Children in Hospital, 7 Exton Street, London SE1 8VE. (01-261 1738)

National Deaf Children's Society, 31 Gloucester Place, London W1H 4EA. (01-486 3251)

National Eczema Society, Mary Ward House, 5–7 Tavistock Place, London WC1. (01-387 9681)

National Society for Autistic Children, 1a Golders Green Road, London NW11. (01-453 4375)

National Society for Brain Damaged Children, Honorary Secretary, 35 Larchmere Drive, Hall C, Birmingham.

National Society for Mentally Handicapped Children, 117 Golden Lane, London EC1Y ORT. (01-253 9433)

National Society of Phenylketonuria and Allied Disorders, 6 Rawdon Close, Palace Fields, Runcorn, Cheshire. (092-85 65081)

NSPCC, 1 Riding House Street, London W1.

Royal National Institute for the Blind, 224 Great Portland Street, London W1N 6AA. (01-388 1266)

Royal National Institute for the Deaf, 105 Gower Street, London WC1E 6BR. (01-387 8033)

Scottish Council for Spastics, 22 Corstorphine Road, Edinburgh. (031-337 2804)

Scottish Society for the Mentally Handicapped, 69 West Regent Street, Glasgow G2 2AN. (041-331 1551)

Scottish Spina Bifida Association, 190 Queensferry Road, Edinburgh. (031-332 0743)

Spastics Society, 12 Park Crescent, London W1N 4EQ. (01-636 5020)

Toy Libraries Association, Seabrooke House, Wyllyots Manor, Darkes Lane, Potters Bar, Hertfordshire EN6 5HC. (0707 44571)

Appendix 4
Normal values and conversion tables

(Normal values)

Haemoglobin
Newborn   16.6 g/dl
Age 12 years $\begin{cases} 13.8\,\text{g/dl girls} \\ 14.0\,\text{g/dl boys} \end{cases}$

Red blood cells
Newborn $4.5–5.0 \times 10^6/\text{mm}^3$
Age 12 years $4.2–5.4 \times 10^6/\text{mm}^3$

White blood cells
Newborn $16–20 \times 10^3/\text{mm}^3$
Age 12 years $4–12 \times 10^3/\text{mm}^3$

Platelets
$200–500 \times 10^3/\text{mm}^3$

Sedimentation rate (Westergren)
2–10 mm/h

Total protein   5.2–7.8 g/dl
Albumin   3.5–5.0 g/dl
Globulin   1.7–2.8 g/dl
Fibrinogen   0.2–0.4 g/dl
Bilirubin   0.1–0.5 mg/dl

Serum electrolyte

Sodium	136–143 mmol/litre
Potassium	4.1–5.6 mmol/litre
Chloride	98–106 mmol/litre
Bicarbonate	21–25 mmol/litre
Urea	2.5–6.7 mmol/litre

Blood sugar

Serum glucose (fasting)	3.4 to 5.6 mmol/litre

Cerebrospinal fluid

Pressure	50–150 mmH_2O (7.5–20 kPa)
Sugar	3.9–4.8 mmol/litre
Total protein	10–30 mg/dl
Cells	<5 lymphocytes/mm^3

Urine (24-hour content)

Protein (total)	30–50 mg
Urea	200–500 mg/kg body weight/day

Average blood pressures

	Systolic		Diastolic	
Age	(mm Hg)	kPa	(mm Hg)	(kPa)
Birth	65–95	8.5–13	30–60	4–8
5 years	80–110	11–15	45–65	6–8.5
10 years	90–120	12–16	50–70	7–9

Normal distribution of body fluids—as percentage of body weight

	Premature infants	F.T. infants	Children	Adults
Body water (%)	75–80	70–75	60–70	55–60
Extracellular (blood and between cells)	40–50	35–40	30–50	20
Intracellular	30–50	35	30–50	40

Normal daily water loss—infants and children

	Urine (ml)	Stool (ml)	Skin (ml)	Total (ml)
Infant (2–10 kg)	200–500	25–40	80–300	800–840
Child (10–40 kg)	500–800	40–100	300–600	840–1500

Index